Advance Praise for *The Art and Science of Compassion, A Primer*

"Well-written, deeply personal and scientifically grounded, this book provides strong physiological, psychological, and ethical reasons why cultivating compassion is essential—and provides a thoughtful roadmap for promoting compassion in healthcare and in all of life."

—**Ron Epstein, MD**, author of *Attending: Medicine, Mindfulness, and Humanity*

"Dr. Agnes Wong, a highly distinguished physician and exceptional researcher at the University of Toronto, has written an absolutely uplifting masterpiece about meaning, compassionate care, and the universal journey that all healers must take to sustain their inner being and nobility of purpose. This book is partly her journey to a deeper state of being that places compassionate care in its rightful place in the healing art; it is also a fabulous scientific presentation of the practice and impact of compassionate care on patients and on one's own flourishing as a physician. This is a book that touches the soul and should be read by every medical student or clinician worldwide as they reflect on what it means to really succeed in their "whole selves" as healers and human beings."

—**Stephen G. Post, PhD**, Director, Center for Medical Humanities, Compassionate Care and Bioethics; Professor of Family, Population, and Preventive Medicine, Stony Brook University

"Compassion and empathy are traits that make us human, and as Dr. Wong shows, these qualities can be developed, encouraged, and cultivated. In our struggling world, we need this awareness as never before. The future of our species likely depends on it. This book is an example of how science and spirituality can come together in a brilliant synthesis."

—**Larry Dossey, MD**, author of *One Mind: How Our Individual Mind Is Part of a Greater Consciousness and Why It Matters*

The Art and Science of Compassion, A Primer

Reflections of a Physician-Chaplain

AGNES M.F. WONG, MD, PHD, FRCSC

Professor of Ophthalmology, Neurology, and Psychology
University of Toronto
Toronto, Ontario
Canada

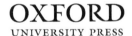

OXFORD
UNIVERSITY PRESS

OXFORD
UNIVERSITY PRESS

Oxford University Press is a department of the University of Oxford. It furthers
the University's objective of excellence in research, scholarship, and education
by publishing worldwide. Oxford is a registered trade mark of Oxford University
Press in the UK and certain other countries.

Published in the United States of America by Oxford University Press
198 Madison Avenue, New York, NY 10016, United States of America.

Library of Congress Cataloging-in-Publication Data
Names: Wong, Agnes M.F., 1968– author.
Title: The art and science of compassion, a primer : reflections of
a physician-chaplain / Agnes M.F. Wong.
Description: New York, NY : Oxford University Press, [2021] |
Includes bibliographical references and index.
Identifiers: LCCN 2020030314 (print) | LCCN 2020030315 (ebook) |
ISBN 9780197551387 (paperback) | ISBN 9780197551400 (epub) |
ISBN 9780197551417 (online)
Subjects: MESH: Empathy | Compassion Fatigue—psychology |
Professional-Patient Relations | Attitude of Health Personnel
Classification: LCC BF575.E55 (print) | LCC BF575.E55 (ebook) |
NLM BF 575.E55 | DDC 152.4/1—dc23
LC record available at https://lccn.loc.gov/2020030314
LC ebook record available at https://lccn.loc.gov/2020030315

DOI: 10.1093/med/9780197551387.001.0001

This material is not intended to be, and should not be considered, a substitute for medical or
other professional advice. Treatment for the conditions described in this material is highly
dependent on the individual circumstances. And, while this material is designed to offer
accurate information with respect to the subject matter covered and to be current as of the
time it was written, research and knowledge about medical and health issues is constantly
evolving and dose schedules for medications are being revised continually, with new side
effects recognized and accounted for regularly. Readers must therefore always check the
product information and clinical procedures with the most up-to-date published product
information and data sheets provided by the manufacturers and the most recent codes of
conduct and safety regulation. The publisher and the authors make no representations or
warranties to readers, express or implied, as to the accuracy or completeness of this material.
Without limiting the foregoing, the publisher and the authors make no representations or
warranties as to the accuracy or efficacy of the drug dosages mentioned in the material. The
authors and the publisher do not accept, and expressly disclaim, any responsibility for any
liability, loss, or risk that may be claimed or incurred as a consequence of the use and/or
application of any of the contents of this material.

5 7 9 8 6

Printed by Marquis, Canada

To Joseph and Esther, for giving me this precious life;
James and Stephen, for bringing much joy and a new dimension to
my being;
Bill, for your love, trust, and unwavering support as we travel this
journey together;
and
Roshi Joan, for showing me the way to a wholehearted practice in
this world.

Contents

Foreword

Roshi Joan Halifax

At a science conference in India, His Holiness the Dalai Lama noted that "Compassion is not religious business; it is human business. It is not a luxury . . . it is essential for human survival." He later wrote, "However capable and skilful an individual may be, left alone, he or she will not survive. However vigorous and independent one may feel during the most prosperous periods of life, when one is sick or very young or very old, one must depend on the support of others. . . . I believe that at every level of society—familial, tribal, national, and international—the key to a happier and more successful world is the growth of compassion."

We cannot say with certainty whether compassion is genetic, instinctual, intentional, cultural, or socially prescribed. However, we have learned from scientific research that compassion enhances the welfare of those who receive it and also benefits those who give it. Compassion also benefits those who observe an act of compassion.

Over my years of caring for dying people, I came to see that compassionate presence can reduce the anxiety dying people experience and can also have a positive effect on those who serve others who are suffering.

Years ago, my student Dr. Gary Pasternak, the medical director of Mission Hospice in San Mateo, California, and a long-term meditator, sent me an email that moved me deeply. It exemplified the qualities that I have come to value in a physician. He wrote,

> I'm up late admitting patients to the inpatient hospice unit. Just when I think I'm too old for these late nights without sleep, a person in all their rawness, vulnerability, and pain lays before me and as my hands explore the deep wounds in her chest and my ears open to her words, my heart cracks open once again. . . . And this night a sweet 36-year-old woman with her wildly catastrophic breast cancer speaks of

her acceptance and her hope for her children, and she speaks with such authenticity and authority. And her acceptance comes to me as the deepest humility a person can experience and then again, once again, I remember why I stay up these late nights and put myself in the company of the dying.

Dr. Pasternak's words reflect respect, humility, care, and courage. He was able, in the midst of distractions and sleep deprivation, to slow down and open to the reality of life, suffering, pain, and death. For me, this is compassion: the ability to turn toward the truth of suffering with concern, care, and equanimity and with the wish to relieve that suffering.

I believe that compassion is central to us being fully human. It is also a key to reducing systemic oppression and nurturing a culture of respect, civility, and belonging. It is an experience that makes cultures, organizations, and humans successful. To help us understand the necessity of compassion, science is making a strong case for its benefits and the importance of compassion for our survival and fundamental health. This book addresses why and how compassion is a necessity in the medical workplace. To this end, I want to give a bit of background on how compassion found its way into neuroscience laboratories.

In the summer of 2011, a group of scientists, scholars, and contemplatives gathered in Berlin in the studio of Icelandic/Danish artist Olafur Eliasson to explore approaches appropriate to training in compassion as well as important questions related to neuroscience research into compassion. The invitation was offered by a leader in neuroscience research at the Max Planck Institute in Leipzig.

The vision behind this meeting was that compassion was an essential feature in personal and social well-being, but one that had not been adequately mapped neurally, nor had training protocols been developed that would serve in secular settings. The thought was that neuroscience research into compassion might yield important insights into how to train others in compassion and would also point to the value of compassion in medicine, education, and other areas of life.

As we know, compassion is often associated with religion. It is also believed by some to be potentially unhealthy and the cause of distress in those who manifest it. This Berlin meeting was supported in the hopes that important research endeavours related to compassion in Europe, the United States, and Asia would eventually be pursued.

Before the meeting in Berlin, neuroscience research on compassion was in its early stages. Relatively small number of meditation adepts participated as research subjects in the laboratories of neuroscience and social psychology so that scientists could map the neural substrates of compassion and assess its psychological and physiological effects. More recent research projects have involved explorations of immune response in relation to compassion and, as well, compassion's effects on longevity. Because there seems to be a deficit of it in our society, including in the field of medicine, research on compassion has taken a quantum leap in recent years, including in the laboratories of the Max Planck Institute in Germany and Keck Laboratory in Madison, Wisconsin.

In order to research compassion and ultimately to develop training approaches in compassion in relation to medicine and other disciplines, one must have a clear understanding of how compassion is structured and operates. To this end, the meeting in Berlin was an important step by contemplatives, social psychologists, and neuroscientists in exploring the process and structure of compassion.

For many decades, I myself have been engaged in the study of compassion by delving deeply into the literature on compassion, analyzing my own experience as a contemplative practitioner, receiving traditional teachings on compassion from Buddhist masters, working with neuroscientists and social psychologists on research questions related to compassion, being present for the profound suffering encountered by dying people and by those in the prison system, and, most importantly, training professional caregivers and patients in approaches to compassion.

These combined experiences led me to question how we define compassion in our culture and, as well, to question the effectiveness of how we train others in compassion. To this end, I developed a heuristic map of compassion and a training intervention in cultivating compassion in the process of interacting with others. The map is called the A.B.I.D.E. model and the intervention is called G.R.A.C.E., a mnemonic for: *g*athering attention, *r*ecalling intention, *a*ttuning first to self and then to other, *c*onsidering what will serve, and *e*ngaging and ending. Now G.R.A.C.E. has been taught in many parts of the world in clinical settings, including in Asia, Europe, and the Americas.

I was fortunate that Dr. Agnes Wong, my student and a brilliant clinician, brought her keen mind to explore how compassion could serve clinicians. This book is the result of her direct experience as a clinician, her observations of the challenges clinicians face in giving care to others, and her finely tuned synthesis of compassion research, including my work in compassion.

Compassion has been loosely defined as the emotion one experiences when feeling concern for another's suffering and desiring to enhance that person's welfare. Compassion has two main aspects: the affective feeling of caring for one who is suffering and the motivation to relieve that suffering. As Dr. Wong has noted, however, compassion is a much more nuanced experience, a process that is contingent and emergent. It is grounded in interrelationality and is an experience of mutuality that is reciprocal and asymmetrical. Thus, compassion is possibly not a discrete feature per se, but an emergent and contingent process that is fundamentally context-sensitive.

If this is the case, then training others in the medical field in the cultivation of compassion necessitates that one discovers the processes that nourish and enhance compassion. It is also an exploration of what can sustain clinicians as they face the suffering of their patients and, as well, the suffering of their colleagues and themselves. Dr. Wong's precise work reflects these questions and gives a clear picture of how the instantiation of compassion in medical training will serve both clinicians and patients. Her book is an important, timely, and challenging work that will open many doors for those who read it.

Roshi Joan Halifax, PhD
Abbot, Upaya Zen Center and Institute,
Santa Fe, New Mexico

Foreword

Gregory L. Fricchione

In this very fine book, Dr. Agnes M.F. Wong—a well-known neuro-ophthalmologist and neuroscientist—melds her personal story with an important message for patients, family members, caregivers, and society at large that emanates from her unique perspective as a physician, scientist, and Buddhist chaplain. After suffering a severe bout with hearing loss and the distress of severe tinnitus, she stopped to take stock of her life in the midst of deep melancholy. She found a new appraisal of what matters and discovered that this meaningful place where the better angels of our nature reside in a spirit of awareness of the present moment infused with compassion and loving kindness, can present all of us with a springboard to healing and indeed to flourishing. Dr. Wong lays out the present-day neuroscientific hypothesis about why mindfulness meditation—the product of single point focus attention and non-judgmental open awareness—can change brain structure and function and importantly, "set the stage for compassion/loving-kindness training by modulating attentional resources (in the attention networks), regulating emotion processing and control (in the limbic system), and altering self-referential processing (in the default mode network)." She proceeds to argue cogently about the desperate need we have as individuals and as society itself to nurture the practice of mindfulness and compassion and then she tells us the good news that there are protocols available that do just that. In essence, she writes:

> To build inner compassion, we need to shift from the threat system to activate the affiliative system. By intentionally slowing down, mindfulness training is particularly valuable in allowing us to choose to respond differently. By activating the affiliative system, we are better able to *think* and to *behave* in more compassionate ways.

It is a common misconception in the public that meditation is all about learning to detach from the world. I once asked a friend of mine, the Buddhist monk and psychologist, Dr. Lobsang Rapgay, about whether the Buddha had non-attachment as his goal for developing classical mindfulness. I recall him saying that the Buddha was trying to find a way that would strengthen our ability to be present with those who are suffering and to offer them relief in solace and succor. So, meditation is ultimately about enhancing one's capacity to attach in compassion to those who are suffering.

Dr. Wong knows this and expresses this great wisdom very wisely in this book.

Gregory L. Fricchione, MD
Associate Chief of Psychiatry
Massachusetts General Hospital
Mind Body Medical Professor of Psychiatry
Harvard Medical School
Boston, MA

Preface

What Is This Book About?

Compassion is a core value in healthcare. A recent survey shows that 85% of patients and 91% of doctors value compassion, making it the most important principle in healthcare.[1] However, terms like "compassion," "empathy," and "sympathy" have been used interchangeably in common parlance, and their definitions vary in the literature. This semantic and conceptual confusion has important implications for clinical practice, medical education, and research. In addition, while medical schools offer courses on communication skills, patient–physician relationships, and social determinants of health, compassion is inconsistently taught, valued, and measured,[2] partly because of the lack of a standard curriculum that covers the full gamut of this construct, from conceptual to experiential.

This book is designed as a short, "all-in-one" introductory text that covers the full spectrum of compassion, from the evolutional, biological, behavioural, and psychological, to the social, philosophical, and spiritual. Written with busy trainees, clinicians, and educators in mind, it aims to address the following questions concisely: What is compassion? Is it an emotion, a motivation, or is it multidimensional? Is it innate or a trainable skill? What do different scientific disciplines, including neuroscience, tell us about compassion? Why is "compassion fatigue" a misnomer? What are the obstacles to compassion? Why are burnout, moral suffering, and bullying so rampant in healthcare? Why does compassion decrease during medical training? And, finally, what does it take to cultivate compassion? It is my hope that by providing readers with a solid conceptual framework, the materials presented here will inspire, reinforce, and integrate with the experiential component of compassion that requires diligent cultivation, training, and practice.

Why Did I Write This Book?

I am a physician, scientist, and educator. I work in a tertiary/quaternary pediatric hospital and am a professor in a major academic centre in North America. I once thought that I lived a very fulfilling life: providing the best care to children and their families through direct patient work, generating exciting new medical knowledge through research, and nurturing new generations of physicians and scientists through teaching, as well as serving my colleagues, hospital, university, and the larger healthcare system through various leadership positions.

With my drive, determination, and work ethic, I ascended the academic ladder rapidly, being promoted from assistant, to associate, and then to full professor in fewer than 10 years. I was named a highly coveted endowed Chair at the relatively young age of 40. When I was 45, I became the Chief of Ophthalmology in my hospital and the Vice Chair of Research in my university department. I held multiple prestigious research grants simultaneously for many years, published extensively in top journals in my field, and directed a large laboratory that hired many scientists, engineers, technicians, and students. I travelled around the world on a regular basis, giving keynote speeches and named lectureships, along with being a visiting professor. I received numerous accolades for my research and teaching endeavours. I felt that I was truly blessed because I would not have accomplished all these without the unyielding support of a loving husband and two adorable sons. Many would say I had reached the pinnacle of success as a physician-scientist while at the same time achieving a very fine work–life balance.

But these accomplishments were not enough. I strived to advance upward by pursuing a degree in Master of Business Administration while managing a full workload. Then, something completely unexpected happened. I developed a hearing loss in one ear, 4 years ago, at age 48. The worst part of it was a constant, 24/7, non-stop ringing in my ear. I could not rest, I could not sleep, I could not have a moment of peace and quiet. I was treated with steroid injections into my ear. I was also put on oral steroids. Not only did they not help, I developed suicidal thoughts which frightened me to the core. When all Western treatment options were exhausted, my doctor covertly told me that he did not want to see me anymore. I felt abandoned, desperate, and hopeless inside. But, on the outside, I put on a brave face and continued to carry out all of my duties, pretending that I could endure all of these challenges with my usual determination and perseverance.

As I suffered deeply inside, I began to see clearly all the sufferings around me. I realized that, despite many successes, our satisfaction seems to be short-lived—very soon it diminishes, and we find ourselves wanting more. At times, we become unhappy because we don't get what we want, or we get what we don't want, or we worry about things not going our way. As I looked around, I felt deeply the stress that my co-workers experience every day from an excessive workload, the agony that we face when making complex and difficult decisions, the moral distress that we witness in the workplace, the tugging at our hearts from our family and relationships as we juggle multiple competing demands, and, ultimately, the suffering that we all have to confront through sickness, old age, and the inevitable demise of our loved ones and eventually our own self.

I started to see more and more vividly the cycles of stress and anxiety that we all encounter, as well as how my own reactivity contributes to these cycles of negativity that affect not only myself but also everyone around me. I began to realize clearly that our well-being does not come from achieving, acquiring, and accumulating. While there is nothing inherently wrong with the rewards that come from hard work, the pitfalls of success come when maintaining these privileges— in my case, a successful medical practice, prestigious academic titles and honours, an esteemed social status, big house, nice car, exotic vacations—become an obligation. At a certain point in time, the pursuit of material possessions, pleasures, praise, and recognition makes life feel hollow. Without awareness and the courage to look deeply or make changes, we may work harder and accumulate more only to find that the happiness and deep fulfilment that we long for remain elusive.

I began to realize that true happiness can come only by examining what's inside, by investigating the relationship between the external world and our inner self, and by changing our habitual patterns in response to our thoughts, feelings, and emotions. After a very long period of reflection—the dark night of my soul*—I decided to pursue

---

* This phrase originates from a poem by St. John of the Cross (1542–1591), a Spanish Carmelite monk and mystic, whose best known work *Noche Oscura del Alma* is translated as "The Dark Night of the Soul."

a different path and do the unthinkable. I stepped down from all the leadership positions before completing my terms. I closed my laboratory. I turned part-time. However, my heart was torn because all of these radical changes were incompatible with my deeply ingrained ambition, competitiveness, and perfectionism. Going through these changes felt like a career suicide, an existential crisis, a mini-death. I kept thinking: What will people think of me? Am I disappointing my hospital staff? How could I be so irresponsible by abandoning many long-time employees whose livelihoods depend on me? Will I ever be trusted again? Am I setting a bad example for my kids and trainees by being a "quitter"? Are the many years of training and the experiences that I have accumulated to finally become a highly specialized expert going to waste? What will be the financial implications? Confronting these questions was painful, heart-rending, and frightening. Unknown to me, my identity, self-worth, and sense of purpose had been wrapped up completely with my roles, titles, and external validation. I asked myself: Who am I *really*, and what should I do next? I knew deep inside that I must commit to my decision no matter how raw, excruciating, and harrowing the process was.

I began by looking at what I enjoyed most. I realized that what has brought me the most joy was meeting people, listening to them, and serving them in whatever way I could. I also recognized that I have been increasingly drawn to the spiritual needs of the dying, having witnessed and been immersed in some truly life-changing, genuinely human, and amazingly enriching experiences while caring for my dying father, mother-in-law, and mentors. At the same time, I have been practising mindfulness for several years, which has helped me to be stronger, calmer, and more opened to new perspectives. I wanted to delve deeper into its roots that originate in Buddhist traditions. Out of these considerations, I resolved to pursue chaplaincy training with Roshi Joan Halifax,* so that I could hone my skills to serve others and explore how to care for the dying while at the same time deepen my spiritual practice.

---

* The term "Roshi" is a respectful honorific to a precious teacher or a master in the Zen tradition.

Chaplaincy training has been a deeply healing and transformative experience. I now realize that I must touch deeply into my own pain and sorrow so that I can look clearly into the underlying causes of the inherent unsatisfactoriness of our conventional lives. From a visceral appreciation of the universality of suffering, a deep motivation was aroused in me: to lead an awakened life with integrity, courage, and wholehearted practice, to alleviate the miseries of all beings, and to touch the true nature of reality. Learning to embrace not knowing, to bear witness to the joys and pain of life, and to discern what is the most skilful action at each moment has been challenging and yet, paradoxically, deeply grounding and nourishing. I can now see acutely that my earlier notion of service, though noble and well-meant, was based on many previously hidden, naïve, and incomplete assumptions and orientations. It was based on the concept of "fixing" what is broken and "helping" what is weak from a position of being better and stronger, rather than coming from a deep inner place of humility to serve life as whole.* I also notice, despite the best intention to serve, how quickly, easily, and furtively my ego slips in for its own gratification.

Chaplaincy training has brought me to many unanticipated, uncharted, yet remarkable territories. Working as a hospice volunteer in the community, I came to know a "dying" young woman with a malignant brain tumour. She had been given less than a year but continued to live for another decade. I feel that I have come full circle. As a neuro-ophthalmologist, I see patients with brain tumours regularly, monitoring their visual and neurologic functions. I have rarely paused, if ever, to imagine what living a life with multiple handicaps, uncertainties, and imminent threats of death feels like. At the same time, the strength, resilience, and wisdom this young woman revealed have given me a new appreciation of the mystery and sacredness of living and dying.

Through serendipity, I have also become a volunteer in a prison, working with inmates on a weekly, one-on-one basis. It is truly an

* I learned the differences between helping, fixing, and serving from Dr. Rachel Naomi Remen who wrote: "Helping, fixing, and serving represent three different ways of seeing life. When you help, you see life as weak. When you fix, you see life as broken. When you serve, you see life as whole. Fixing and helping may be the work of the ego, and service the work of the soul" (*Shambhala Sun*, September 1999).

eye-opening experience beyond my wildest imagination. I have become a witness to the most unimaginable, horrendous, and unbearably painful life circumstances that these men have endured from a very young age. I am astonished to notice a common theme among these men: extreme poverty, discrimination, physical and sexual abuses, alcohol and drug addictions, mental illnesses, psychological traumas, and violence, as well as brain and other physical injuries. Moreover, these adverse conditions seem to span generations. I also see how these men are forgotten by society, incarcerated in prison with its culture of subordination, without freedom, without having their simple needs or basic human rights met. They constantly continue to face physical and sexual violence, cruelty, injustice, loneliness, fear, and worse. Their experiences have made me realize that I have lived a privileged life, cocooned and ignorant of how different it could have been. How could I not bring my presence, my willingness to listen, and my companionship to these men who have never had the opportunities that I have taken for granted?

With these poignant exposures to life's adversity, I realized that I need to cultivate a deeper compassion and skilful means before I can truly serve others. Therefore, I decided to take a deep dive to study compassion in earnest for my chaplaincy thesis, combining my longstanding interests in psychology, biology, neuroscience, and social science with my curiosity to explore Buddhist teachings in greater depth. When I first encountered the ideal of *bodhisattvas*— enlightened beings who are motivated to end all sufferings until all are liberated—I was completely enthralled. It was as if the ordeal of my hearing loss (which has since resolved) had cracked open my heart to hear the cries of the world, dissolving my personal boundary beyond time and space. When I first came across the idea of the "great compassion"—a non-referential, boundless compassion that becomes one's *raison d'être* not only to practise wholeheartedly, but also to pursue intellectual understanding to penetrate into the ultimate truth—I was moved to tears. I now realize that my interests in the sciences and my love for reading and writing, as well as my zeal for teaching, are not necessarily self-centered pursuits that hinder the path to awakening. On the contrary, I can realign my interests with a deep aspiration and intention to benefit all others. The results of this recognition and exploration on the sciences of compassion led to the first half of the present book.

As I was nearing the completion of the thesis, I began to understand a main reason why I decided to make such a drastic change in my career: my disillusionment with the healthcare system. As a leader, I envisioned and attempted to build a more compassionate culture in the workplace where everyone—doctors, nurses, staff, administrators, and all others—comes together not only to serve patients and their families, but also one another, so that everyone can live a purposeful, fulfilling, and authentic life. Although there were some small successes, I was also met with much skepticism, cynicism, or silent acquiescence to the status quo. I pondered deeply inside and explored why I hit many roadblocks by reaching out to colleagues, other healthcare professionals, and caregivers to learn from their experiences. I researched and investigated why there is so much distress, burnout, and suffering in the healthcare world. I now have a fuller understanding of the hurdles that caregivers face, as well as some skilful ways to cultivate a compassionate and flourishing life, which I discuss in the second half of this book.

It is with great joy that I share this book with you. Whether you are a medical student, physician-in-training, practising doctor, nurse, social worker, therapist, chaplain, hospice worker, caregiver, volunteer, or someone who wants to live a compassionate and flourishing life, I sincerely hope that this book will encourage you to cultivate compassion as a skilful means to serve others and look more deeply into your own life. Individually and collectively, we can transform healthcare into a kinder, more caring system, as well as build a gentler, more just society that is so needed in this burning world.

References

1. Patients favor compassion, clinician empathy over low doc costs. 2018. https://patientengagementhit.com/news/patients-favor-compassion-clinician-empathy-over-low-doc-costs
2. Lown BA, Chou CL, Clark WD, et al. Caring attitudes in medical education: Perceptions of deans and curriculum leaders. *J Gen Intern Med.* 2007;22(11):1514–1522.

1
What Are Empathy and Compassion?
A Western Perspective

Introduction

As a young aspiring student, I wrote in my medical school application that I wanted to become a doctor in order to help others through science and compassion. When I went into medical school in the early 1990s, I soon became immersed in a curriculum that placed strong emphasis on scientific and technical excellence. I studied the latest advances in basic and clinical sciences, the different diseases and their processes, as well as the myriad of tests, drugs, and procedures. Very little, if any, curriculum time was dedicated to the cultivation of compassion—in fact, I can't recall a single instance when the word "compassion" was mentioned.

While compassion is an important quality of a good doctor, there seems to be an implicit assumption that we cannot develop compassion in the same way that we acquire technical knowledge and skills. There also seems to be a widespread belief that compassion is soft and incompatible with science or that you can be compassionate at your own peril because compassion is limited, heavy, and fatiguing. It is perhaps not surprising that when we become residents, being thrown into the deep end with a constant flow of patients while having a gruelling work schedule, we find ourselves exhausted and our intention to serve with compassion a distant ideal. When we become independent practitioners, after being conditioned to believe that compassion is limited, we may offer compassionate care guardedly, perhaps unconsciously trying to shield ourselves from increased patient demands, time pressures, and the "compassion fatigue" that plague healthcare today. But does it have to be this way?

The purpose of this book is to lay out succinctly the scientific evidence showing that compassion is both innate and trainable. We will see that we already have within ourselves a natural store of deep compassion and wisdom. There are also many ways to cultivate compassion to support the practice of medicine and the art of caregiving in general. The training described in this book draws on both contemplative and scientific disciplines to help us develop cognitive, attentional, affective, and somatic skills that are critical for the cultivation of compassion. Compassion not only benefits those we serve, produces better patient care, and improves our healthcare system; it is also a boundless source of energy, resilience, and wellness so that, as we serve, we can also enjoy a truly flourishing life.

In this chapter, we begin by examining the definitions of "empathy" and "compassion." Although these two terms are distinct, they have been used interchangeably, which has helped perpetuate the common misconception that compassion is finite and emotionally draining. We will also look at their evolution to gain an appreciation of how humans became successful as a species because of our nurturing, altruistic, and compassionate attributes that have evolved over millions of years.

Empathy

The word "empathy" has its origin in the ancient Greek *empatheia*, which literally means *en* (in) *pathos* (passion). The philosopher Robert Vischer was the first to use the German expression *einfühlung*, meaning "feeling into," which was later translated into the English word "empathy" by Edward Bradford Titchener, one of the founding fathers of the discipline of psychology.[1]

In addition to the notion of *feeling into* the experiences of another (an *affective* component), contemporary scientific usage of the term "empathy" also encompasses a *cognitive* component. Also called *perspective-taking* or *mentalizing*, this cognitive component involves a differentiation between the experience of another and that of the self. According to Singer and colleagues,[2] empathy is a human capacity to share and understand others' emotions without confusing them with one's own feelings. In other words, we empathize with others when we vicariously share their affective state, while at the same time we are aware that our response is elicited by their emotion. As such, empathy can be conceptualized as having four components: (1) an affective sharing, (2) an isomorphism of this affective sharing (i.e., sharing the same emotional state as the other), (3) a mental representation of the other's affective state, and (4) a top-down discrimination of self from other.[3] From this definition, we can see an evolution of our understanding of empathy from an original, more automatic "feeling into" the experiences of another (i.e., emotional empathy—the first two components of the concept) to the cognitive modulation of affective sharing through a top-down differentiation of self from other (i.e., cognitive empathy—the last two components).

In addition to a distinction between emotional and cognitive empathy, empathy can lead to two divergent responses: empathic distress and empathic concern.[4] *Empathic distress* is an aversive and self-oriented emotional response to others' suffering. It is often associated with withdrawal behaviour to protect oneself from negative emotional experiences when the self–other distinction becomes blurred. Empathic distress is especially relevant for healthcare workers as they are often and repeatedly exposed to others' suffering, which can result in emotional exhaustion and burnout. Fortunately, empathy does not inevitably lead to empathic distress. Through awareness and training, empathy can be transformed skilfully into *empathic concern*, an other-focused, more adaptive and positive emotion and a motivation that primes compassion,[5–7] a topic that I discuss in the next section.

The origin of empathy can be traced back to well beyond the emergence of human and non-human primates. Its earliest vestiges can be found more than a hundred million years ago in primitive mammalian species including elephants, dolphins, and whales, in the forms of motor mimicry, emotional contagion, and pre-concern.[8] From dogs howling to the distant cries of coyotes (mimicry), to toddlers crying when another toddler cries in a nursery (emotional contagion), to the seemingly spontaneous approaching behaviour of a young rhesus monkey to another which is injured (pre-concern), there are abundant behavioural examples in the natural world that are considered precursors of empathy. Using "Russian dolls" as a model, the Dutch primatologist and ethologist Frans de Waal suggested that emotional connection is the innermost core around which empathy evolves and is constructed (Figure 1.1).[8] Bodily and emotional connection—the innermost core—induces in the subject an emotional state that is similar to that of the object (i.e., state-matching between subject and object). As prefrontal lobe functioning and self–other distinction increase in higher species, sympathetic concern and perspective-taking—the doll's middle and outer layers—evolve. The hard-wired innermost emotional core, however, remains fundamentally linked to the outer layers and generates somatic/emotional perception and action (perception–action mechanism). According to de Waal, empathy has evolved and been selected for its prosocial, protective, and survival value.[8,9] In particular, empathy is likely to have emerged as a result of increased parental care as a means to improve offspring survival in species with a so-called *K-selected life history pattern* (long individual life span, small litter size, immaturity at birth with long dependence on

THE RUSSIAN DOLLS MODEL OF EMPATHY LAYERS

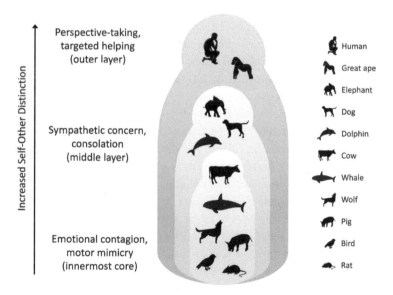

Figure 1.1 The Russian dolls model showing the layered nature of empathy as proposed by Frans de Waal.[8]

parental care, low offspring mortality) rather than in an *r-selected spe-cies* with the opposite life history pattern.[10,11]

Compassion

The term "compassion" derives from the Latin word *compati*, meaning literally *to suffer with*. Considered one of the most cherished of virtues among all major religious traditions, the practice of compassion has been described in the Vedic Upanishads (written between 500 and 800 BCE) and the early Buddhist scriptures (500 BCE) in ancient India. Later, compassion emerged in the Islamic Qur'an in the recitations of Rahman,[12] in the ideals of Tzedakah in the Jewish Torah, in the medical texts of the Babylonians,[13] in the Bible of the Christian faith, and in the oral history of Native Americans. Today, compassion is advocated in many religions and is epitomized by many figures, including the 14th Dalai Lama, Mother Theresa, Desmond Tutu, and Nelson Mandela, to name just a few.

The definition of compassion, however, varies according to cultural context, as do the functions and qualities attributed to it. For example, Aristotle argued that compassion arises only when the other's suffering is serious, when we have some sense of that suffering, and when the other deserves our compassion. There have been diverging views about whether compassion is an emotion,[14] motivation,[15] or a multidimensional construct.[16] Most contemplative traditions as well as contemporary scientific disciplines, however, generally converge on a definition of compassion that is multifaceted. For example, Geshe Thupten Jinpa, translator for the 14th Dalai Lama, defines compassion as a multidimensional process comprised of four key components: (1) an awareness of suffering (cognitive component), (2) sympathetic concern related to being emotionally moved by suffering (affective component), (3) a wish to see the relief of that suffering (intentional component), and (4) a responsiveness or readiness to help relieve that suffering (motivational component).[16] Similarly, emotions researcher Paul Ekman suggests four dimensions of compassion: (1) empathic compassion (being in touch with the feelings of others who suffer), (2) action compassion (taking action to alleviate suffering),

(3) concerned compassion (based on a motivation for helping), and (4) aspirational compassion (linked to a more cognitive desire to develop compassion).[17]

For the purpose of this book, I will use a definition of compassion that is consistent with Eastern traditions and is also accepted by most social cognitive neuroscientists and social psychologists: compassion is a sensitivity to the suffering of self and others with a commitment to alleviating and preventing it.[15] There are three implicit components in this definition: (1) a (brief) affective empathy—one briefly "feels into" the negative experience of another; (2) a cognitive labeling of the experience as suffering by the other, including the ability to take perspective of the other and to engage in self–other differentiation; and (3) a desire or readiness to alleviate that suffering. Importantly, it is this third component that differentiates compassion from empathy; that is, unlike empathy, compassion directs one's attention to help others. It involves top-down processing, such that there is a more immediate self–other differentiation and a shift to recognize suffering as common to all humanity. It is also interesting to note that, for the third component, one does not have to actually help others but only to have the desire to do so.

As discussed in the previous section, empathy can lead to two responses: empathic distress and empathic concern (which primes compassion). We can now see that a critical component of these differential responses is the success of self–other differentiation. In empathic distress, there is an over-involvement or over-identification of the self in the perception of another's suffering, producing self-focused, aversive, and avoidant behaviour. In contrast, in empathic concern, after an initial brief affective empathy, one quickly shifts and differentiates oneself from the other to allow for other-focused, prosocial, helping motivations and behaviours to emerge.

With the difference between empathic distress and empathic concern (compassion) in mind, it is important to note here that the term "compassion fatigue" is a misnomer.[18-21] First coined by Carla Joinson in 1992, it describes a unique form of burnout in nurses that arises from a variety of stressors and results in a "loss of the ability to nurture."[22] Later, Figley described it as a "caregiver's reduced capacity or interest in being empathic or bearing the suffering of clients."[23] It is a "manifestation of succumbing to the demands of client care over self-care of those who provide the care of clients as a professional."[24] The characteristics of distress, over-identification with the suffering of others, and the lack of self-care that these authors suggested are consistent with empathic distress. "Empathic fatigue" (or "empathic distress") is therefore a better term than "compassion fatigue" to describe this unique form of burnout, although the latter is still commonly used in the literature. This distinction is not only one of semantics, but it is crucial because (1) numerous studies have demonstrated the physical and psychological benefits of compassion on caregivers (see Chapter 3); (2) advances in neurosciences have shown that the brain networks that mediate empathic distress and compassion are distinct (see Chapter 5); (3) there is an inverse relationship between compassion and burnout; that is, high compassion is protective against burnout, whereas low compassion increases the risk of burnout (see Chapter 7); (4) the lack of self-care—a major cause of empathic fatigue and burnout—can be remedied by cultivating inner compassion (see Chapter 7); and (5) the wish or motivation for others to be free from suffering, a feature that distinguishes compassion from empathy, makes compassion a wellspring of indefatigable energy for caregivers, even in situations when no action can be taken to produce useful results.[20,21]

Compassion is related to three other concepts: altruism, sympathy, and pity. Compassion is differentiated from *altruism* in that altruism spans the gamut from a mere motivational state to alleviate others' suffering[25] to the *actual* engagement in helping behaviours.[26] Both compassion and altruism are thus associated with prosocial motivations. "Sympathy" derives from the Latin word *sympatheia*, meaning literally *feeling (patheia) together (sym)*. Although compassion and sympathy are often used interchangeably in everyday language,[9] sympathy lacks the desire to help others that is found more typically in the term compassion. "Pity," derived from the Latin word *pietas* or *pious*, not only suggests a feeling of sorrow or distress over other's suffering, but also involves a subtle feeling of superiority over the person who is suffering.[14]

From an evolutionary perspective, compassion requires higher order executive functions that are found only in primates, and it is thus a much more recent phenomenon than empathy. While non-human primates may exhibit "compassionate" behaviours, these behaviours are distinct from those in humans. For example, chimpanzees and bonobos, which shared common ancestry with humans around 6–8 million years ago, are known to provide *fleeting* help to those able to reciprocate the favour, and they engage in extended care for *infants*.[8] What is unique in ancient hominids is their provision of care to *adults* and for *extended* periods of time.[27] Indeed, anthropological evidence from remains of skulls, teeth, and bones dating back more than a million years ago indicates that early humans with congenital deformities, illnesses, and injuries sometimes survived for decades, which would not have been possible without the extended care of others.[28] The evolution of compassion generally is believed to result from extreme climate variability more than 5 millions years ago[29] that exerted selective pressure on our ancestors to move into collaborative hunting, food-sharing, and collective parenting.[30] Such social collaboration, in turn, led to the emergence of emotional capacities including prosociality.[27] These capabilities enabled our ancestors to risk their own well-being to protect others from predators, to forgo immediate gratification to share food with others, and to invest in another's well-being when the person being helped is a stranger who gives the benefactor no immediate benefit.[28] Interestingly, this period paralleled a time when the human brain became larger and more complex with the development of the neocortex, the significance of which will be discussed in Chapter 3.

Inner Compassion

Compassion can flow in three directions: to others, from others, and to self. Self-compassion, a Western psychological construct popularized by researcher Kristin Neff,[31] is defined as compassion for oneself, or a sensitivity to one's own suffering and a desire to alleviate that suffering.[12] Neff proposed that self-compassion is composed of three components: (1) *self-kindness*—feelings of loving-kindness toward one's self, similar to what a compassionate person would feel toward another, together with the desire to alleviate any suffering one may feel rather than being harshly self-critical; (2) *mindfulness*—a sense of balance or equanimity, as well as nonjudgment and receptivity toward one's thoughts, feelings, and experiences, rather than over-identifying with them; and (3) *common humanity*—a sense of shared membership with the rest of humanity, with all the accompanying joys, trials, and tribulations, rather than seeing them as separate and isolating.[32] Distinct from the long-established Western focus on self-esteem, self-compassion has been shown to be an important indicator for psychological well-being.[32,33] Indeed, Neff suggested that self-esteem is based on downward social comparison and judgment of self-worth and is often associated with narcissism, self-centredness, reduced concern for others, out-group discrimination, and even hostility and violence.[33] Evolutionarily, self-compassion is traceable to the self-grooming behaviour of primates.[9]

Survival of the Kindest

Like many who grow up in a competitive, meritocratic culture, I used to believe that Charles Darwin's (1809–1882) "survival of the fittest" is a law of nature and that successes are guaranteed for the brightest and hardest working—assuming unconsciously that everyone has equal opportunities—with compassion almost an afterthought. This "law" seems to run counter to the evidence we have reviewed here showing that humans have evolved to become more collaborative and compassionate in our quest to thrive. As I was doing my research, I came to realize that many have misunderstood Darwin's view on natural selection by equating it with "survival of the fittest." In his book *On the Origin of Species* published in 1859,[34] Darwin proposed natural selection as a process to explain how species evolve over time. In this process, genotypic variations that increase a species' chances of survival are preserved and passed to the next generation, so that eventually only individuals with favourable traits that are most adaptable to their particular environment survive. It is worth noting that Darwin did not coin the phrase "survival of the fittest." Instead, it was the social Darwinist Herbert Spencer (1820–1903) who first coined this phrase, 7 years after Darwin's publication of his theory. Borrowing

Darwin's concept on biology, Spencer expanded and applied it to other disciplines, including economic, social, and political philosophies, to justify cut-throat economic competition, eugenics, and racism.[35] Since then, "survival of the fittest" has been used to suggest that creatures are perpetually engaged in a merciless struggle in which only the fittest survive. This adversarial worldview was further popularized by Thomas H. Huxley (1825–1895), known as "Darwin's bulldog," and by the poet Alfred Tennyson (1809–1892) who suggested that nature is "red in tooth and claw."[36] It is revealing to find that, contrary to this cruel, competitive paradigm that is commonly attributed to him, Darwin later wrote about the importance of sympathy (what we would call compassion today) in *Descent of Man* in 1871: "In however complex a manner [sympathy] may have originated, as it is one of high importance to all those animals which aid and defend one another, it will have been increased through natural selection; for those communities, which included the greatest number of the most sympathetic members would flourish best, and rear the greatest number of offspring." He also wrote: "We are impelled to relieve the sufferings of another, in order that our painful feelings may be at the same time relieved."[37] For Darwin, therefore, "sympathy" is not only essential for survival, but is also the foundation of humanity, in which moral concerns contribute to the development of individuals and communities. From this, we can conclude that "survival of the kindest"[38] may be a better description of the origins and journey of humanity. What is perhaps most fascinating is that, even if you don't believe in evolution, many ancient sages, prophets, mystics, logicians, and philosophers arrived at the same conclusion on the universality of compassion. Indeed, the principle of compassion lies at the heart of all religious, ethical, and spiritual traditions, a topic that I will discuss in Chapter 4.

Summary of Key Points

- Empathy and compassion are two distinct concepts. In the simplest sense, empathy is feeling *into* the experiences of another, whereas compassion is feeling *for* another with an additional desire/motivation to alleviate the suffering of the other.

- Empathy has four components: (1) an affective sharing, (2) an isomorphism of this affective sharing (i.e., sharing the same emotional state of the other), (3) a mental representation of the other's affective state, and (4) a top-down discrimination of self from other. The first two components are sometimes called *emotional empathy*, whereas the last two components are called *cognitive empathy*.

- Empathy can lead to two responses, depending on emotion regulation: empathic distress and empathic concern. When emotion is unregulated, empathic distress occurs, which is an aversive and self-oriented emotional response to others' suffering. When emotion is regulated, empathic concern occurs, which is an other-focused, adaptive, positive emotion and motivation. In other words, empathy is often a precursor to and primes compassion when emotion is regulated, but empathy is not compassion.

- Compassion has three components: (1) a (brief) affective empathy—one briefly "feels into" the negative experience of another; (2) a cognitive labeling of the experience as suffering by the other, including the ability to take perspective of the other and to engage in self–other differentiation; and (3) a desire or readiness to alleviate that suffering. It is this third component that additionally differentiates compassion from empathy; that is, unlike empathy, compassion directs one's attention to help others, which may or may not involve actually helping these others.

- "Compassion fatigue" is a misnomer. "Empathic fatigue" is a better term to capture the distress, over-identification with the suffering of others, and the lack of self-care that are characteristics of caring professionals experiencing empathic distress or burnout.

- Compassion is a much more recent evolutional phenomenon than empathy because compassion requires higher order executive functions that are found only in primates.

- Compassion can flow in three directions: to others, from others, and to self.

References

1. Stueber K. Empathy. In: Zalta EN, ed. *The Stanford Encyclopedia of Philosophy.* Stanford, CA: Stanford University; 2017. https://plato.stanford.edu/entries/empathy/

2. de Vignemont F, Singer T. The empathic brain: how, when and why? *Trends Cogn Sci.* 2006;10(10):435–441.

3. Singer T, Lamm C. The social neuroscience of empathy. In: Miller MB, Kingstone A, eds. *Year in Cognitive Neuroscience 2009.* Boston, Mass: Blackwell Pubulication on behalf of the New York Academy of Sciences; 2009:81–95.

4. Vrtička P, Favre P, Singer T. Compassion and the brain. In: Gilbert P, ed. *Compassion: Concepts, Research and Applications.* Oxon, UK: Routledge, Taylor & Francis Group; 2017:135–150.

5. Eisenberg N, Fabes RA, Miller PA, et al. Relation of sympathy and personal distress to pro-social behavior: A multimethod study. *J Pers Soc Psychol.* 1989;57(1):55–66.

6. Batson CD, Fultz J, Schoenrade PA. Distress and empathy: Two qualitatively distinct vicarious emotions with different motivational consequences. *J Pers.* 1987;55(1):19–39.

7. Batson CD, Duncan BD, Ackerman P, Buckley T, Birch K. Is empathic emotion a source of altruistic motivation? *J Pers Soc Psychol.* 1981;40(2):290–302.

8. de Waal FB. Putting the altruism back into altruism: the evolution of empathy. *Annu Rev Psychol.* 2008;59:279–300.

9. de Waal F. *The Age of Empathy.* New York: Three Rivers Press; 2009.

10. MacArthur RH, Wilson EO. *The Theory of Island Biogeography.* Princeton, NJ: Princeton University Press; 1967.

11. Gonzalez-Liencres C, Shamay-Tsoory SG, Brune M. Towards a neuroscience of empathy: Ontogeny, phylogeny, brain mechanisms, context and psychopathology. *Neurosci Biobehav Rev.* 2013;37(8):1537–1548.

12. Stevens L, Woodruff CC. What is this feeling that I have for myself and for others? Contemporary perspectives on empathy, compassion, and self-compassion, and their absence. In: Stevens L, Woodruff CC, eds. *The Neuroscience of Empathy, Compassion, and Self-Compassion.* London: Academic Press, Elsevier; 2018:1–21.

13. Reynolds EH, Wilson JV. Depression and anxiety in Babylon. *J R Soc Med.* 2013;106(12):478–481.

14. Goetz JL, Keltner D, Simon-Thomas E. Compassion: An evolutionary analysis and empirical review. *Psychol Bull.* 2010;136:351–374.

15. Gilbert P. Compassion: Definitions and controversies. In: Gilbert P, ed. *Compassion: Concepts, Research and Applications.* Oxon: Routledge, Taylor & Francis Group; 2017:3–15.

16. Jazaieri H, Lee I, McGonigal K, et al. A randomized controlled trial of compassion cultivation training: Effects on mindfulness, affect, and emotion regulation. *Motiv Emot.* 2013;38:23–35.
17. Ekman P. Moving toward global compassion. 2014. www.paulekman.com
18. Hofmeyer A, Kennedy K, Taylor R. Contesting the term "compassion fatigue": Integrating findings from social neuroscience and self-care research. *Collegian.* 2020;27(2):232–237.
19. Dowling T. Compassion does not fatigue! *Can Vet J.* 2018;59(7):749–750.
20. Ricard M. *Altruism: The Power of Compassion to Change Yourself and the World.* New York: Little, Brown and Company; 2015.
21. Halifax J. *Standing at the Edge.* New York: Martin's Press; 2018.
22. Joinson C. Coping with compassion fatigue. *Nursing.* 1992;22(4):116, 118–119, 120.
23. Figley CR. Introduction. In: Figley CR, ed. *Compassion Fatigue: Secondary Traumatic Stress Disorders from Treating the Traumatized.* New York: Brunner Mazel; 1995:xiii–xxii.
24. Figley CR, Figley KR. Compassion fatigue resilience. In: Seppälä EM, Simon-Thomas E, Brown SL, Worline MC, Cameron CD, Doty J, eds. *The Oxford Handbook of Compassion Science.* New York: Oxford University Press; 2017:387–398.
25. Batson C. *Altruism in Humans.* New York: Oxford University Press; 2011.
26. Monroe KR. *The Heart of Altruism: Perceptions of a Common Humanity.* Princeton, NJ: Princeton University Press; 1996.
27. Spikins P. Prehistoric origins. The compassion of far distant strangers. In: Gilbert P, ed. *Compassion: Concepts, Research and Applications.* Oxon: Routledge, Taylor & Francis Group; 2017:16–30.
28. Haddad GG, Sun Y, Wyman RJ, Xu T. Genetic basis of tolerance to O_2 deprivation in *Drosophila melanogaster. Proc Natl Acad Sci U S A.* 1997;94(20):10809–10812.
29. Potts R, Faith JT. Alternating high and low climate variability: The context of natural selection and speciation in Plio-Pleistocene hominin evolution. *J Hum Evol.* 2015;87:5–20.
30. Domínguez-Rodrigo M, Bunn HT, Mabulla AZP, et al. On meat eating and human evolution: A taphonomic analysis of BK4b (Upper Bed II, Olduvai Gorge, Tanzania), and its bearing on hominin megafaunal consumption. *Quatern Int.* 2014;322:129–152.
31. Neff K. *Self-Compassion: The Proven Power of Being Kind to Yourself.* New York: William Morrow; 2015.
32. Neff KD. The development and validation of a scale to measure self-compassion. *Self Identity.* 2003;2:223–250.
33. Neff K. Self-compassion: An alternative conceptualization of a healthy attitude toward oneself. *Self Identity.* 2003;2:85–101.

34. Darwin C. *On the Origin of Species*. West Sussex, UK: John Wiley & Sons; 2020.
35. Burdett C. Post Darwin: Social darwinism, degeneration, eugenics. British Library. https://www.bl.uk/romantics-and-victorians/articles/post-darwin-social-darwinism-degeneration-eugenics
36. Doty J. Preface. In: Seppälä EM, Simon-Thomas E, Brown SL, Worline MC, Cameron CD, Doty J, eds. *The Oxford Handbook of Compassion Science*. New York: Oxford University Press; 2017:xxi–xxii.
37. Darwin C. *The Descent of Man*. New York: Penguin Classics; 2004.
38. Keltner D. *Born to be Good: The Science of a Meaningful Life*. New York: W. W. Norton; 2009.

2
Is Compassion Innate?
A Physiological Perspective

According to Charles Darwin, emotions are best understood as evolved and adaptive processes that facilitate communication and connection.[1] Of all human emotions and behaviours, compassion could be considered the best exemplar of Darwin's claim. Natural selection has created pressure for humans to evolve from an individualistic "self-preservative" system into a prosocial "species-preservative" system.[2,3] The self-preservative system, developed early in evolutionary history, focuses on survival by avoiding harm and securing resources such as food and shelter. It is based on a sense of self versus other. The more recently evolved species-preservative system, on the other hand, is based on a more inclusive sense of the self and interconnectedness. It evolved from maternal instincts to protect and promote the welfare of vulnerable offspring, leading to support for clan members and, ultimately, the development of biological subsystems that support a compassion that extends to all beings and the planet.

This species-preservative system can be conceptualized as comprising three interrelated biological subsystems: (1) the autonomic nervous system, specifically the newly evolved ventral myelinated vagus nerve, which allows moment-to-moment fine-tuning of physiological and emotional regulation to promote social engagement behaviours; (2) the neuroendocrine system, specifically the hormones and neurotransmitters vasopressin and oxytocin, which facilitate kinship and clan emotional bonding; and (3) the central nervous system, specifically an enlarged neocortex (including the prefrontal and cingulate cortices), which allows improved self–other differentiation and the ability to understand another's emotion. In this chapter, I explore the first two subsystems. The role of the central nervous system in mediating compassion will be discussed in Chapter 5.

The Autonomic Nervous System

The autonomic nervous system is comprised of two antagonistic subsystems, the *sympathetic* and *parasympathetic nervous systems*. In general, the autonomic nervous system prioritizes threat detection via the sympathetic nervous system, which catalyzes a cascade of autonomic changes aimed at self-protection (fight-or-flight response). In nonthreatening contexts, the parasympathetic nervous system, in particular the ventral myelinated vagus nerve, produces calm states that encourage affiliation and bonding. The American scientist Stephen Porges proposed the polyvagal theory (Figure 2.1),[4,5] which states that there are two functionally distinct branches of the vagus nerve: (1) the dorsal branch, which is unmyelinated, more primitive, and is responsible for immobilization behaviours when threatened; and (2) the ventral branch, which is myelinated, more recently evolved, and is responsible for inhibiting the sympathetic fight-or-flight response in service of social affiliative behaviours. In mammals, the myelinated ventral branch facilitates proximity seeking at birth, as opposed to the disbursement found in most reptiles. It enhances the experience of soothing and safeness, facilitates connection and engagement, and

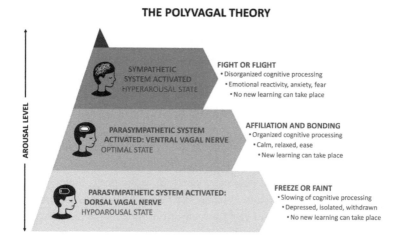

Figure 2.1 The polyvagal theory and the autonomic nervous system.[4,5]

promotes caretaking and bonding.[4,5] Indeed, the ventral myelinated vagus nerve innervates facial muscles that are critical to social communication and engagement behaviours, including looking, listening, facial expression, vocalizing, filtering of low-frequency sounds for the discrimination of human voices from background sounds, and head gestures. Higher vagal tone, as measured by increased heart rate variability, represents activation of the parasympathetic nervous system.[6] Empirical studies in humans have shown a link between higher vagal tone and a compassionate disposition.[7] A link between higher vagal tone and situational compassion in response to witnessing another suffer is also evident.[8] Porges further suggested that the ventral myelinated vagus nerve, together with the release of oxytocin (discussed later), may have coopted defensive systems involved in freezing when threatened for immobilization during nursing, reproduction, and social bonding.[4]

In conjunction with greater vagal activation in the autonomic nervous system, the experience of compassion is also accompanied by increased activation in the periaqueductal gray.[9] Importantly, the periaqueductal gray projects to those part of the brainstem where the ventral vagus nerve originates,[10] indicating that these two structures may communicate directly with one another. In addition, oxytocin levels are associated with vagal activity. The anatomical and observed associations between the ventral myelinated vagus nerve, periaqueductal gray, and oxytocin suggest the potential for an integration of hormonal, autonomic, and neural responses during compassion.

The Neuroendocrine System

Classically, hormones are chemicals produced by specialized glands that regulate the activity of different bodily tissues through blood circulation. However, hormones can also function as neurotransmitters in the central nervous system. An example is the neuropeptide vasopressin (also called *arginine vasopressin* or *antidiuretic hormone*), which is produced in the hypothalamus. As a hormone, vasopressin is known for its role in reducing urine output by stimulating the kidneys to reabsorb water. Interestingly, discoveries over the past decades indicate that vasopressin can also behave like a neurotransmitter to promote prosocial behaviours. In animal studies, vasopressin has been shown to mediate male affiliative, pair-bonding, and paternal behaviour.[11,12] In humans, vasopressin is linked to increased threat responses in men but increased affiliative responses in women.[13] It also increases reciprocal cooperative behaviours in humans, with increased activation of affiliative brain areas (including the bed nucleus of the stria terminalis, lateral septum, and stria terminalis) and decreased activation of arousal areas in the autonomic nervous system.[14] A vasopressin gene receptor (V1a) has been associated with altruism and social interactions.[15,16]

Another neuropeptide that has been studied extensively and plays a crucial role in prosocial behaviour is oxytocin. Like vasopressin, oxytocin is primarily synthesized in the hypothalamus. As a hormone, it is known for its role in childbirth and lactation (Figure 2.2). As a neurotransmitter, it exerts profound effects on areas of the brain that directly modulate social behaviours, including empathy and compassion.[17] For example, central oxytocin promotes caring motivation[18,19] by virtue of its facilitating interactions with the reward-seeking mesolimbic dopaminergic system.[20] It fosters prosocial caregiving by reducing avoidance and the fear of novelty through a reduction of amygdala activation, a neural circuitry involved in aversive behaviours.[21] At the same time, it enhances acceptance and other-oriented behaviours[21] through increased activation in regions involved in empathic responses (the insula and inferior frontal gyrus).[22] In addition, oxytocin is associated with feelings of safeness and belonging that are critical for the expression of compassion.[23] Importantly, it heightens one's ability to understand another's perspective[24] while maintaining self–other distinction,[25] which are essential elements of empathy and compassion.

However, oxytocin fosters prosocial behaviours only to certain targets, such as kin or members from an in-group (an exclusive group of people with a shared interest or identity),[27] indicating that the underlying motivation and social context in which oxytocin functions are critical. Indeed, oxytocin can increase maternal aggression when offspring are threatened, as well as increase one's hostility to individuals perceived as members of an out-group.[28] Oxytocin creates intergroup

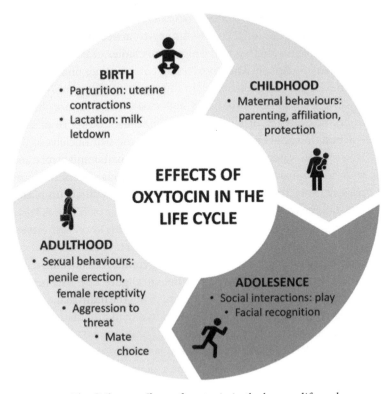

Figure 2.2 The different effects of oxytocin in the human life cycle. Redrawn from Lee et al.[26]

bias by promoting in-group favouritism and out-group discrimination. Contrary to popular belief, oxytocin is not a generalized "love hormone" or "cuddle chemical" as it plays a role in the generation of intergroup conflict and violence.

Behavioural Genetics

The most commonly studied gene associated with prosociality is the oxytocin receptor gene OXTR, which has a polymorphism (OXTR rs53576) localized in a single copy of human chromosome 3.[29] People who have the G allele (vs. A allele) of OXTR rs53576 tend to be more sensitive to socioemotional cues in the environment, displaying more positive social interactions and empathic behaviours.[30–32] They also exhibit greater empathy when processing emotionally salient features or when seeing others in distress.[33] In addition to OXTR rs53576, other oxytocin-related genes (rs1042778 and rs6449182 polymorphisms) have been linked to socially affiliative emotions and more positive interactions in social relationships.[34,35]

However, as discussed earlier, oxytocin has a complex relationship to both empathic and compassionate prosocial behaviours and to negative social actions such as withdrawal and intergroup biases. Some studies have shown that carriers of the G allele of OXTR rs53576 are more sensitive to negative social stressors, with lower self-esteem and diminished perceived meaningfulness in response to social ostracism or exclusion.[36] Those with a G/G genotype show heightened sympathetic cardiac reactivity to psychological stressors[37] and greater autonomic arousal when perceiving harm to others, indicating that oxytocin receptor variation plays an important role in modulating physiological reactions to affective experiences.[32]

To reconcile the apparent discrepancies of positive and negative social outcomes from oxytocin receptor gene expressions, a model of gene–environment interactions has been proposed.[38] The model suggests that carriers of oxytocin-related genes may be more socially sensitive to environmental cues in different context. When they are exposed to nonthreatening stimuli that provide them with opportunities for affiliation, they are more inclined to express empathic and compassionate behaviours. However, when confronted with potentially threatening cues, they are more prone to exhibit emotions and behaviours that are negative in valence, including social withdrawal, diminished self-esteem, and emotional dysregulation. For example, G/G genotype carriers are at risk for increased emotional dysregulation and enhanced disorganized adult attachment style after being exposed to an environment in which the carriers experienced severe abuse in childhood.[39]

Similarly, a gene–culture interactions model has been suggested to explain the cultural differences often observed in gene–environment interactions. Cultural background is an important factor in shaping what people with certain genetic predispositions consider a relevant social cue.[38] For example, among distressed American participants, those with G allele reported seeking more emotional social support, whereas Korean participants did not differ significantly by genotype. These findings indicate that OXTR rs53576 is sensitive to input from cultural norms regarding social behaviours.[40]

Physiological Benefits of Compassion

While researching on the biological basis of compassion, I found it equally fascinating to discover that the physiological mechanisms that underlie the expression of compassion elicit similar effects on those who receive it. Recipients of compassion not only experience a sense warmth and kindness, but the dynamic between their sympathetic and parasympathetic nervous systems also changes, enhancing their health and well-being. For example, isolation and loneliness have reached an all-time high in the West, with nearly half of Americans surveyed reported feeling lonely or left out, a problem that is particularly severe in older adults.[41,42] This is alarming because there is robust evidence showing that social isolation is a major risk factor for mortality, rivalling the effects of other well-known risk factors such as cigarette smoking, obesity, high blood pressure, and high cholesterol level.[43-47] One explanation for the adverse effect seen in social isolation is psychosocial stress, which leads to activation of the sympathetic nervous system (fight-or-flight response) and a concomitant rise in circulating cortisol. Cortisol is a hormone known to play important roles in chronic inflammation[48] and immune response suppression,[49-51] as well as in the development of cardiovascular disease and stroke.[52,53] Sympathetic arousal also leads to the release of the hormone adrenaline, which can cause anxiety, apprehensiveness, restlessness, tremor, weakness, and respiratory difficulties. Indeed, excessive adrenaline can provoke a curious, potentially fatal condition called *Takotsubo cardiomyopathy*.[54] Also known as *stress-induced myopathy* or "broken heart syndrome," this disease is usually the result of severe emotional stress such as the loss of a loved one. The heart muscles weaken, causing the left ventricle to bulge out like a balloon or an octopus trap (*tako-tsubo* in Japanese), reducing the heart's ability to pump blood out to the rest of the body.[54]

Compassion counteracts the adverse effects of sympathetic arousal by activating the parasympathetic nervous system, including increased vagal tone,[55] and by the release of the neurotransmitter oxytocin.[56] Recipients of compassion had decreased respiratory and heart rates, as well as increased heart rate variability—all indicators of "relaxation response" from parasympathetic activation.[57,58] Interestingly, these effects were greater when compassion was received through non-verbal than verbal communication.[58] A "warm touch" between married partners led to reductions in sympathetic activation as measured by decreased blood pressure and increased oxytocin secretion.[56] Social support also lowered cardiovascular reactivity to acute stressors.[59,60]

In addition, compassion reduces pain perception, likely through the release of endogenous opioids such as endorphins, which reduce the brain's sensitivity to pain. For example, empathic touch from a trusted partner elicited lower subjective pain scores.[61] Interestingly, physiological coupling occurred between partners: high partner empathy was not only associated with a decrease in pain perception by the recipient, but the partner's respiration and heart rates also increased correspondingly, becoming in sync with those of the recipient.[62] Compassion also enhances resilience when under threat. Receiving support from relational partners attenuated both subjective distress and brain activity in a network associated with emotional and behavioral threat, including areas that are responsible for salience detection, vigilance, and regulation of self-control.[63,64]

Finally, the speed of wound healing is also affected by compassion. Supportive couples who were subjected to experimental blister wounds healed faster compared to those who exhibited hostile marital behaviours. In addition, their plasma inflammatory cytokines (interleukin 6 and tumor necrosis factor-alpha), which inhibit wound healing, were significantly less than those found in acrimonious couples.[65] Faster wound healing was also found to be correlated with higher oxytocin and vasopressin levels in supportive couples.[66]

As we can see in this chapter, compassion is innate and is built into our biological system. However, it could be obscured by the adversity of individual experiences, motivations, social context, and social conditioning which teach us who is or is not deserving of our compassion. It is therefore crucial that we develop resilience against life's adversity, undo our often unconscious conditioning, and investigate our many unexamined biases in order to cultivate a compassionate life that excludes no one. How we connect—how we care or fail to care—can impact one another in significant ways. In the next chapter, I will discuss the psychological basis of compassion. We will see that compassion not only benefits the recipients, but it also has a powerful impact on the physical and mental health of the givers.

Summary of Key Points

- Three biological subsystems subserve affiliative and compassionate behaviours: the autonomic nervous system, neuroendocrine system, and central nervous system.
- The autonomic nervous system consists of the sympathetic and parasympathetic nervous systems. The sympathetic nervous system prioritizes threat detection, leads to hyperarousal, and initiates the fight-or-flight response. According to the polyvagal theory, the vagus nerve, which is part of the parasympathetic nervous system, consists of two branches: dorsal and ventral. The dorsal branch is responsible for immobilization (freeze or faint) behaviours when threatened, leading to a hypoarousal state. The newly evolved ventral branch, in contrast, allows for emotional regulation, leads to an optimal arousal state, and promotes social affiliative behaviours.
- The neuroendocrine system, through the neuropeptides vasopressin and oxytocin, facilitates kinship and emotional bonding. Synthesized in the hypothalamus, both neuropeptides function as a hormone (antidiuresis for vasopressin, and parturition and lactation for oxytocin) and as a neurotransmitter to enhance prosocial, affiliative behaviours.
- Contrary to popular belief, oxytocin is not a general "love hormone" because it also plays a role in the generation of intergroup conflict and violence. In this regard, the underlying motivation of the individuals, social context, gene–environment interactions,

and gene-culture interactions are all critical in determining whether oxytocin promotes positive versus negative social actions.
• The physiological mechanisms that underlie the expression of compassion also elicit similar effects on those who receive it. Recipients of compassion have increased parasympathetic nervous system activation and enhanced release of oxytocin and vasopressin. They exhibit reduced cardiovascular reactivity, decreased pain perception, increased resilience to threat, and faster wound healing.

References

1. Darwin C, Ekman P, Prodger P. *The Expression of the Emotions in Man and Animals*. New York: Oxford University Press; 1998.
2. MacLean PD. *The Triune Brain in Evolution: Role in Paleocerebral Functions*. New York: Plenum Press; 1990.
3. Henry JP, Wang S. Effects of early stress on adult affiliative behavior. *Psychoneuroendocrinology*. 1998;23(8):863–875.
4. Porges SW. The polyvagal theory: Phylogenetic substrates of a social nervous system. *Int J Psychophysiol*. 2001;42(2):123–146.
5. Porges SW. The polyvagal perspective. *Biol Psychol*. 2007;74(2):116–143.
6. Laborde S, Mosley E, Thayer JF. Heart rate variability and cardiac vagal tone in psychophysiological research: Recommendations for experiment planning, data analysis, and data reporting. *Front Psychol*. 2017;8:213.
7. Oveis C, Cohen AB, Gruber J, Shiota MN, Haidt J, Keltner D. Resting respiratory sinus arrhythmia is associated with tonic positive emotionality. *Emotion*. 2009;9(2):265–270.
8. Eisenberg N, Fabes RA, Schaller M, et al. Personality and socialization correlates of vicarious emotional responding. *J Pers Soc Psychol*. 1991;61(3):459–470.
9. Simon-Thomas ER, Godzik J, Castle E, et al. An fMRI study of caring vs self-focus during induced compassion and pride. *Soc Cogn Affect Neurosci*. 2012;7(6):635–648.
10. Farkas E, Jansen AS, Loewy AD. Periaqueductal gray matter projection to vagal preganglionic neurons and the nucleus tractus solitarius. *Brain Res*. 1997;764(1–2):257–261.
11. Winslow JT, Hastings N, Carter CS, Harbaugh CR, Insel TR. A role for central vasopressin in pair bonding in monogamous prairie voles. *Nature*. 1993;365(6446):545–548.

12. Insel TR. The challenge of translation in social neuroscience: A review of oxytocin, vasopressin, and affiliative behavior. *Neuron.* 2010;65(6):768–779.

13. Thompson RR, George K, Walton JC, Orr SP, Benson J. Sex-specific influences of vasopressin on human social communication. *Proc Natl Acad Sci U S A.* 2006;103(20):7889–7894.

14. Rilling JK, DeMarco AC, Hackett PD, et al. Effects of intranasal oxytocin and vasopressin on cooperative behavior and associated brain activity in men. *Psychoneuroendocrinology.* 2012;37(4):447–461.

15. Ebstein RP, Knafo A, Mankuta D, Chew SH, Lai PS. The contributions of oxytocin and vasopressin pathway genes to human behavior. *Horm Behav.* 2012;61(3):359–379.

16. Israel S, Lerer E, Shalev I, et al. Molecular genetic studies of the arginine vasopressin 1a receptor (AVPR1a) and the oxytocin receptor (OXTR) in human behaviour: From autism to altruism with some notes in between. *Prog Brain Res.* 2008;170:435–449.

17. Colonnello V, Petrocchi N, Heinrichs M. The psychobiological foundation of prosocial relationships: The role of oxytocin in daily social exchanges. In: Gilbert P, ed. *Compassion: Concepts, Research and Applications.* Oxon, UK: Routledge, Taylor & Francis Group; 2017:105–119.

18. Meyer-Lindenberg A, Domes G, Kirsch P, Heinrichs M. Oxytocin and vasopressin in the human brain: Social neuropeptides for translational medicine. *Nat Rev Neurosci.* 2011;12(9):524–538.

19. Rilling JK. The neural and hormonal bases of human parental care. *Neuropsychologia.* 2013;51:731–747.

20. Feldman R. Oxytocin and social affiliation in humans. *Horm Behav.* 2012;61:380–391.

21. Carter CS. Neuroendocrine perspectives on social attachment and love. *Psychoneuroendocrinology.* 1998;23:779–818.

22. Riem MM, Bakermans-Kranenburg MJ, Pieper S, et al. Oxytocin modulates amygdala, insula, and inferior frontal gyrus responses to infant crying: A randomized controlled trial. *Biol Psychiatry.* 2011;70(3):291–297.

23. Buchheim A, Heinrichs M, George C, et al. Oxytocin enhances the experience of attachment security. *Psychoneuroendocrinology.* 2009;34(9):1417–1422.

24. Shahrestani S, Kemp AH, Guastella AJ. The impact of a single administration of intranasal oxytocin on the recognition of basic emotions in humans: A meta-analysis. *Neuropsychopharmacology.* 2013;38(10):1929–1936.

25. Colonnello V, Chen FS, Panksepp J, Heinrichs M. Oxytocin sharpens self-other perceptual boundary. *Psychoneuroendocrinology.* 2013;38(12):2996–3002.

26. Lee HJ, Macbeth AH, Pagani JH, Young WS, 3rd. Oxytocin: The great facilitator of life. *Prog Neurobiol.* 2009;88(2):127–151.

27. Gilbert P. The origins and nature of compassion focused therapy. *Br J Clin Psychol.* 2014;53(1):6–41.

28. Schneider B, Gonzalez-Roma V, Ostroff C, West MA. Organizational climate and culture: Reflections on the history of the constructs in the Journal of Applied Psychology. *J Appl Psychol.* 2017;102(3):468–482.

29. Gimpl G, Fahrenholz F. The oxytocin receptor system: Structure, function, and regulation. *Physiol Rev.* 2001;81(2):629–683.

30. Baron-Cohen S, Wheelwright S, Hill J, Raste Y, Plumb I. The "Reading the Mind in the Eyes" test revised version: A study with normal adults, and adults with Asperger syndrome or high-functioning autism. *J Child Psychol Psychiatry.* 2001;42(2):241–251.

31. Rodrigues SM, Saslow LR, Garcia N, John OP, Keltner D. Oxytocin receptor genetic variation relates to empathy and stress reactivity in humans. *Proc Natl Acad Sci U S A.* 2009;106(50):21437–21441.

32. Smith KE, Porges EC, Norman GJ, Connelly JJ, Decety J. Oxytocin receptor gene variation predicts empathic concern and autonomic arousal while perceiving harm to others. *Soc Neurosci.* 2014;9(1):1–9.

33. Tost H, Kolachana B, Hakimi S, et al. A common allele in the oxytocin receptor gene (OXTR) impacts prosocial temperament and human hypothalamic-limbic structure and function. *Proc Natl Acad Sci U S A.* 2010;107(31):13936–13941.

34. Creswell KG, Wright AG, Troxel WM, Ferrell RE, Flory JD, Manuck SB. OXTR polymorphism predicts social relationships through its effects on social temperament. *Soc Cogn Affect Neurosci.* 2015;10(6):869–876.

35. Algoe SB, Way BM. Evidence for a role of the oxytocin system, indexed by genetic variation in CD38, in the social bonding effects of expressed gratitude. *Soc Cogn Affect Neurosci.* 2014;9(12):1855–1861.

36. McQuaid RJ, McInnis OA, Matheson K, Anisman H. Distress of ostracism: Oxytocin receptor gene polymorphism confers sensitivity to social exclusion. *Soc Cogn Affect Neurosci.* 2015;10(8):1153–1159.

37. Norman GJ, Hawkley L, Luhmann M, et al. Variation in the oxytocin receptor gene influences neurocardiac reactivity to social stress and HPA function: A population based study. *Horm Behav.* 2012;61(1):134–139.

38. Birkett M, Sasaki J. Why does it feel so good to care for others and for myself? Neuroendocrinology and prosocial behavior. In: Stevens L, Woodruff CC, eds. *The Neuroscience of Empathy, Compassion, and Self-Compassion.* London: Academic Press, Elsevier; 2018:189–211.

39. Bradley B, Westen D, Mercer KB, et al. Association between childhood maltreatment and adult emotional dysregulation in a low-income, urban, African American sample: Moderation by oxytocin receptor gene. *Dev Psychopathol.* 2011;23(2):439–452.

40. Kim HS, Sherman DK, Sasaki JY, et al. Culture, distress, and oxytocin receptor polymorphism (OXTR) interact to influence emotional support seeking. *Proc Natl Acad Sci U S A.* 2010;107(36):15717–15721.

41. Cigna. US Lonliness Index. *Survey of 20,000 Americans Examining Behaviors Driving Loneliness in the United States.* 2018. https://www.multivu.com/players/English/8294451-cigna-us-loneliness-survey/docs/IndexReport_1524069371598-173525450.pdf

42. Cudjoe TKM, Roth DL, Szanton SL, Wolff JL, Boyd CM, Thorpe RJ. The epidemiology of social isolation: National health and aging trends study. *J Gerontol B Psychol Sci Soc Sci.* 2020;75(1):107–113.

43. House JS, Landis KR, Umberson D. Social relationships and health. *Science.* 1988;241(4865):540–545.

44. Holt-Lunstad J, Smith TB, Layton JB. Social relationships and mortality risk: A meta-analytic review. *PLoS Med.* 2010;7(7):e1000316.

45. Holt-Lunstad J, Smith TB, Baker M, Harris T, Stephenson D. Loneliness and social isolation as risk factors for mortality: A meta-analytic review. *Perspect Psychol Sci.* 2015;10(2):227–237.

46. Rico-Uribe LA, Caballero FF, Martin-Maria N, Cabello M, Ayuso-Mateos JL, Miret M. Association of loneliness with all-cause mortality: A meta-analysis. *PLoS One.* 2018;13(1):e0190033.

47. Perissinotto CM, Stijacic Cenzer I, Covinsky KE. Loneliness in older persons: A predictor of functional decline and death. *Arch Intern Med.* 2012;172(14):1078–1083.

48. Cole SW, Hawkley LC, Arevalo JM, Sung CY, Rose RM, Cacioppo JT. Social regulation of gene expression in human leukocytes. *Genome Biol.* 2007;8(9):R189.

49. Pressman SD, Cohen S, Miller GE, Barkin A, Rabin BS, Treanor JJ. Loneliness, social network size, and immune response to influenza vaccination in college freshmen. *Health Psychol.* 2005;24(3):297–306.

50. Cohen S, Doyle WJ, Skoner DP, Rabin BS, Gwaltney JM, Jr. Social ties and susceptibility to the common cold. *JAMA.* 1997;277(24):1940–1944.

51. Kiecolt-Glaser JK, Marucha PT, Malarkey WB, Mercado AM, Glaser R. Slowing of wound healing by psychological stress. *Lancet.* 1995;346(8984):1194–1196.

52. Hawkley LC, Thisted RA, Masi CM, Cacioppo JT. Loneliness predicts increased blood pressure: 5-year cross-lagged analyses in middle-aged and older adults. *Psychol Aging.* 2010;25(1):132–141.

53. Valtorta NK, Kanaan M, Gilbody S, Ronzi S, Hanratty B. Loneliness and social isolation as risk factors for coronary heart disease and stroke: Systematic review and meta-analysis of longitudinal observational studies. *Heart.* 2016;102(13):1009–1016.

54. Dawson DK. Acute stress-induced (takotsubo) cardiomyopathy. *Heart.* 2018;104(2):96–102.

55. Kok BE, Coffey KA, Cohn MA, et al. How positive emotions build physical health: Perceived positive social connections account for the upward spiral between positive emotions and vagal tone. *Psychol Sci.* 2013;24(7):1123–1132.

56. Holt-Lunstad J, Birmingham WA, Light KC. Influence of a "warm touch" support enhancement intervention among married couples on ambulatory blood pressure, oxytocin, alpha amylase, and cortisol. *Psychosom Med.* 2008;70(9):976–985.

57. Kemper KJ, Shaltout HA. Non-verbal communication of compassion: Measuring psychophysiologic effects. *BMC Complement Altern Med.* 2011;11:132.

58. Shaltout HA, Tooze JA, Rosenberger E, Kemper KJ. Time, touch, and compassion: Effects on autonomic nervous system and well-being. *Explore (NY).* 2012;8(3):177–184.

59. Christenfeld N, Gerin W. Social support and cardiovascular reactivity. *Biomed Pharmacother.* 2000;54(5):251–257.

60. Lepore SJ, Allen KA, Evans GW. Social support lowers cardiovascular reactivity to an acute stressor. *Psychosom Med.* 1993;55(6):518–524.

61. Goldstein P, Shamay-Tsoory SG, Yellinek S, Weissman-Fogel I. Empathy predicts an experimental pain reduction during touch. *J Pain.* 2016;17(10):1049–1057.

62. Goldstein P, Weissman-Fogel I, Shamay-Tsoory SG. The role of touch in regulating inter-partner physiological coupling during empathy for pain. *Sci Rep.* 2017;7(1):3252.

63. Coan JA, Schaefer HS, Davidson RJ. Lending a hand: Social regulation of the neural response to threat. *Psychol Sci.* 2006;17(12):1032–1039.

64. Coan JA, Beckes L, Gonzalez MZ, Maresh EL, Brown CL, Hasselmo K. Relationship status and perceived support in the social regulation of neural responses to threat. *Soc Cogn Affect Neurosci.* 2017;12(10):1574–1583.

65. Kiecolt-Glaser JK, Loving TJ, Stowell JR, et al. Hostile marital interactions, proinflammatory cytokine production, and wound healing. *Arch Gen Psychiatry.* 2005;62(12):1377–1384.

66. Gouin JP, Carter CS, Pournajafi-Nazarloo H, et al. Marital behavior, oxytocin, vasopressin, and wound healing. *Psychoneuroendocrinology.* 2010;35(7):1082–1090.

3

Is Compassion Innate?
A Psychological Perspective

The successful transition from an individualistic self-preservative system to the prosocial species-preservative system operates at a species level. Interestingly, such transition also occurs at an individual level from an evolutional psychology perspective that involves the emotion systems, as well as from a developmental psychology perspective that involves the attachment and caregiving behavioural systems.

Evolutionary Psychology: The Emotion Systems

According to Paul Gilbert, a British clinical psychologist and founder of compassion-focused therapy, there are three basic, innate social motivational systems for interpersonal relating.[1] These three motivational systems are involved in (1) competing and social ranking, to contest for resources such as territory, food, and sexual opportunities, as well as social position and social rank[2]; (2) cooperation and sharing, to become a member of a group or team, with a sense of belonging and connectedness[3] and a shift from "me-ness" to "we-ness"[4]; and (3) caring and nurturing, to care for self and others by exhibiting prosocial,[5,6] altruistic, and helpful behaviours.[7] Indeed, toddlers as young as 18 months exhibit helping behaviours even when the other is a stranger and the child receives no immediate benefit.[8]

In addition to these basic, older motivational systems, three emotion systems have evolved for specific functions: threat/protect (i.e., the threat system), drive/reward (i.e., the drive system), and affiliative/soothing (i.e., the affiliative system) (Figure 3.1). The threat system detects threats, activates defensive strategies, and triggers negative emotions such as anger, anxiety, and disgust.[1] It is now

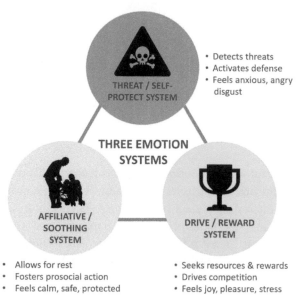

Figure 3.1 The three emotion systems in humans.[1]

known that the threat system is the dominant system and creates a
"negativity bias," so that we pay more attention to and are more likely
to remember negative rather than positive events. This negativity
bias confers an adaptive advantage, so that we are more likely to survive and reproduce.[9] Threat behaviours can be activating, as in fight
and flight, or deactivating, as in defeat, helplessness, and despair.[10]
They are linked to sympathetic nervous system activation and adrenaline production.

The second emotion system, the drive system, provides information on the availability of resources and rewards and activates seeking-
engagement strategies for resource acquisition and achievement.[1]
When linked to seeking out and acquiring resources such as rewards
and skills, the drive system can lead to achievement, success, and pros-
perity. It triggers positive emotions such as joy, fun, excitement, and
pleasure, which are associated with activation of the mesolimbic reward system and dopamine production. However, excessive drive
can lead to unrelenting pursuits of achievement, perfectionism, and

addictive and compulsive behaviours through the dopamine reward-seeking feedback loop.[11,12] In addition, when linked to competition, dominance-seeking, and social positioning, the drive system activates the sympathetic nervous system and adrenaline secretion, causing hyperarousal and stress. This is particularly relevant in our modern culture because an overreliance on achievement and acquiring can increase vulnerability to certain mood disorders, especially when motives are blocked and goals are unmet, thus creating feelings of exhaustion, hopelessness, and burnout.[13]

The third emotion system, the affiliative system, provides information on personal safety, allows for rest and digestion, and enables relative nonaction in the form of contentment and openness.[1] It is linked to positive affects of calming, peace, and contentment—a state of quiescence in which one is not under threat nor in an achieving state of mind, when both the threat and drive systems are inactive. It leads to experiences of warmth, kindness, acceptance, encouragement, support, and affiliation, as well as giving and receiving affection and care from others. The affiliative system is linked to oxytocin, endorphins, and other opioids and the activation of the parasympathetic nervous system.[14]

In addition to these older motivation and emotion systems, about 2 million years ago, a range of cognitive abilities began to emerge in humans as their brains became larger and more complex. The advent of the neocortex enables us to develop mental abilities such as reasoning, reflecting, anticipating, imagining, mentalizing (perspective-taking), ruminating, and creating a sense of self. These new cognitive capacities allow us to become smart, use language and symbols, solve problems, and build technologies. However, a major tradeoff is that humans, unlike other animals, can use these new mental skills to distort the motivation and emotion systems. For example, imagine a zebra on the savannah, where the most stressful event will be to flee from a lion for survival. Once the immediate danger has passed, it will settle and calm down quickly. Humans, on the other hand, can remain traumatized by imagining and ruminating on what *might* have happened. Our capacity to anticipate, imagine, or ruminate can stimulate the threat system continuously, leading to effects that are detrimental to both our physical and mental health.[15] In addition, our intelligence can also be coopted for very destructive purposes, such as building nuclear bombs, using chemical weapons, and inflicting cruelty.[1] Moreover, our newly evolved sense of self can give rise to self-centredness, along with shame, self-criticism, and self-harm. The latter three have been associated with many mental health issues because of constant stimulation of the threat system (see Chapter 6).[16]

We can see from this that the human mind is capable of generating complex and potentially dysfunctional loops among motivations, emotions, and cognition. Fortunately, humans have also evolved motives and emotions for affiliative, caring, and altruistic behaviours to counteract our negative, destructive, and self-serving potentials.[1] By developing our capacity to mindfully access, accept, and direct affiliative motives and emotions—for others and ourselves—we can cultivate skills to shift our mind toward the affiliative system and down-regulate the threat and drive systems. In this way, we can maintain a sense of calmness, well-being, and equanimity.

Developmental Psychology: The Attachment and Caregiving Behavioural Systems

Running alongside the psychology of affiliation and caring is the psychology of attachment. A joint work of British psychoanalyst John Bowlby and American-Canadian psychologist Mary Ainsworth,[17-19] *attachment theory* suggests that there are two behavioural systems, one that governs support-seeking (i.e., the attachment behavioural system) and another that governs support-provision (i.e., the caregiving behavioural system). Drawing on ethological observations, prosociality and compassion are associated with the caregiving behavioural system: an innate system in parents and other caregivers to provide care for young children. This behavioural system is believed to have evolved mainly to complement the attachment behavioural system, which mediates individuals' emotional attachments to their caregivers. Importantly, the interplay between these two systems may account for individual differences in disposition to compassion.

The Attachment Behavioural System

The goal of the attachment system is to attain a subjective sense of security through seeking proximity to a supportive attachment figure. It is made salient by any perceived threat or danger. During infancy, proximity seeking involves crying or crawling toward a caregiver,[20] while in adulthood, it includes establishing contact with or activating mental representations of attachment figures.[21,22] An abiding inner sense of secured attachment based on actual experiences promotes psychological well-being, including having faith in other people's good will, a sense of being loved or understood, and optimistic beliefs about one's ability to handle challenges. However, when attachment figures are not reliably available, an inner sense of secured attachment fails to develop, which leads to a focus on self-protection and secondary strategies that are often inappropriate. These secondary strategies include hyperactivation and deactivation.[23,24] *Hyperactivation* manifests itself as heightened efforts to gain greater proximity, support, and protection while doubting that they can be obtained. *Deactivation*, on the other hand, involves inhibition of proximity-seeking and denial of attachment needs through emotional and cognitive distancing, as well as compulsive self-reliance as the only reliable source of protection. These secondary strategies are reflected in a person's attachment style, which can be measured along two continuous dimensions: *anxiety*, which relies on hyperactivating strategies, and *avoidance*, which relies on deactivating strategies.[25] People who score low on both the anxiety and avoidance dimensions are said to be securely attached.

Although most researchers conceptualize and measure individual differences in attachment as a continuum that varies along the two dimensions of anxiety and avoidance,[26] one popular model combines these two dimensions and categorizes adult attachment into four different styles: secure, anxious, avoidant-dismissive, and avoidant-fearful (Figure 3.2).[27] *Secure* individuals experience a sense of worthiness and believe that others are accepting and responsive. They are confident, resilient, comfortable with intimacy and autonomy, and reciprocal in their relationships with others. Individuals

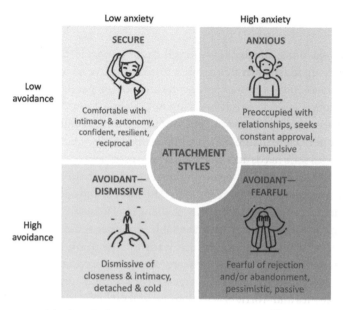

Figure 3.2 The four different attachment styles in adults.[27]

with *anxious attachment style*, on the other hand, feel unworthy and unlovable, combined with a positive evaluation of others. They strive for self-acceptance by seeking constant approval from others and are often preoccupied with relationships. In contrast, people who are highly avoidant comprise the third and fourth categories that differ according to their level of anxiety. Those with *avoidant-dismissive style* experience a sense of worthiness and lovability (low anxiety) combined with a negative disposition toward others. They protect themselves against disappointment by maintaining a sense of independence and invulnerability. They are often detached, cold, and dismissive of closeness and intimacy. Finally, individuals with *avoidant-fearful style* feel unworthy and unlovable (high anxiety) combined with the expectations that others are untrustworthy and rejecting. They protect themselves against anticipated rejection by being pessimistic, passive, and avoiding close involvement with others.[27]

The Caregiving Behavioural System

The goal of the caregiving system is primarily to increase the viability of an individual's own children and family members. Over time, it has evolved to provide protection and support to others who are either momentarily in need or chronically dependent. Effective caregiving is characterized by two qualities: sensitivity (i.e., being attuned to another person's signals of need) and responsiveness (i.e., validating the other person's needs and providing useful assistance), which are at the core of compassion.[28] When children receive sensitive and responsive care, their caregiving system develops under favourable social circumstances, such that loving-kindness, generosity, empathy, and compassion become spontaneous responses to other people's needs. However, when the caregiving system develops under unfavourable circumstances, either because of an absence of supportive attachment figures or when the interactions with the attachment figures engender insecurities and worries, a person is less likely to become empathic or compassionate to another's needs and suffering.[29]

Interplay of the Attachment and Caregiving Systems

Activation of the attachment system can impede the functioning of the caregiving system. For example, from a situational perspective, when people feel threatened, the attachment system is activated such that attention and resources are directed to their own protection and needs rather than those of others.[1] Only when a sense of safety is reinstated can a would-be caregiver provide support to others in need. From a dispositional perspective, people who have more secure attachment are likely to have experienced compassionate role modelling as well as the confidence to support others when they themselves become caregivers. In contrast, people with attachment insecurities are less likely to be responsive to others' needs.[28] For example, those who have attachment anxiety (hyperactivation) tend to fixate on their own unmet attachment needs. In addition, their yearning for closeness may stain their caregiving motivations with self-focused desires for acceptance, which can hamper altruistic helping. Similarly, those who have avoidant attachment (deactivation) are also less likely to help by backing away rather than getting involved, preferring to detach themselves physically, emotionally, and cognitively.

Indeed, numerous studies have confirmed that the interplay between the attachment and caregiving systems is crucial: attachment security makes compassion and altruism more likely.[30-35] People who are relatively secure by disposition, or who are induced to feel secure in a particular context, are less threatened than insecure people by new information, less sensitive to in-group/out-group differences, and more willing to tolerate diversity. They are also more likely to maintain broad humane values, feel compassion toward a suffering other, and engage in altruistic behaviour with the primary goal of benefiting others.

Attachment and Empathy Fatigue in Healthcare

When facing special populations, such as dying patients, people with mental illnesses, victims of terrorism, abused children, and disaster survivors, healthcare professionals are often under extreme stress, which activates their threat/self-protective emotion system and attachment behavioural system. Despite their desire to help others, when these two systems are constantly aroused, their threat response can lead to personal distress, empathy fatigue, and burnout. From a situational perspective, only when a sense of safeness, calmness, and personal agency is present or restored can a caregiver provide compassionate care. From a dispositional perspective, there is also evidence that empathy fatigue is more common in those who have insecure attachment styles, including both anxiety and avoidance.[36-38] Fortunately, research on attachment and caregiving suggests several ways to promote attachment security and effective compassion in caregivers. One is to raise children in ways that strengthen their sense of security, which helps them to become good parents, neighbours, and helpers when they grow up. Another way that is especially useful for adults is to regularly recall times when beneficial support was provided. This recollection may take many forms: visualizing similar situations when a benefactor was present to help; imagining the "perfect nurturer" who offers un-questioning warmth, nonjudgment, and acceptance[39]; remembering acts of kindness exhibited by religious or contemporary figures (Jesus, the Buddha, Muhammad, or Gandhi)[40]; or by looking at pictures of examples of compassion and loving-kindness.[21] These practices may foster compassionate care by increasing one's sense of security and providing one with models of good caregiving.[21]

From this and the previous chapter, we can see that compassion is innate and evolves to enhance the preservation of the human species. This species-preservative strategy leads to the development of physiological and psychological systems that emerge from a basic maternal instinct to protect and nurture vulnerable offspring, to support for clan members, and, ultimately, to a more inclusive sense of the self and interconnectedness that embraces all other beings, the planet, and beyond.

Psychological Benefits of Compassion

In addition to the numerous beneficial physiological effects on the recipients that we discussed in Chapter 2, compassion also improves the psychological health of caregivers. These benefits include improved mood, higher relationship satisfaction, and diminished negative states such as distress, sadness, and guilt.[41-43] Interestingly, giving help is a stronger predictor of better physical and mental health than receiving help from others. For example, giving, but not receiving help, is linked to improved mental well-being and better recovery from bereavement, as well as reduced morbidity and mortality.[44-49] Importantly, the links between helping behaviour and better health are not the results of potential cofounders such as a "helping personality" or a tendency for healthier individuals to help others.[45,50,51] These positive findings also extend to volunteering. Volunteers have lower risk of mortality, better health, and decreased depression levels, as well as slower decline in self-reported health and functioning levels than do nonvolunteers.[52-54]

Informal caregiving (i.e., helping family members and loved ones in need) was once thought to negatively impact caregivers' health[55,56]; however, more recent evidence from better-designed, large-scale prospective studies suggests that informal caregivers enjoy more positive states, including improvements in psychological well-being, health, and longevity.[50,51,57-59] Importantly, the positive effect on longevity holds even when caregivers spent high number of hours in helping.[51,58]

The beneficial effects on caregivers help explain the "helpers' high" that we all have experienced—the uplifting feeling after listening to a friend in need or after doing a good deed or an act of kindness. It also leads us back to an important point I made earlier in Chapter 1. As we can see, compassion in and of itself does not cause fatigue; instead, it enhances the health and well-being of caregivers. On the other hand, empathy fatigue—a form of burnout and empathic distress—is real. It is caused by over-identification with other's suffering, accumulated unaddressed stresses, and self-neglect.[60,61] To alleviate and prevent empathy fatigue and burnout, it is crucial for caregiving professionals to cultivate compassion as an antidote not only for ourselves personally, but also for the ailing healthcare system, a topic that I will discuss in Chapter 7.

Summary of Key Points

- There are three emotion systems: threat/self-protect, drive/reward, and affiliative/soothing.
- The threat system detects threats and triggers negative emotions such as anger, anxiety, and disgust. It creates a "negativity bias" to enhance survival and results in threat behaviours that can be activating (fight and flight) or deactivating (defeat, helplessness, and despair). It is linked to sympathetic nervous system activation and adrenaline production.
- The drive system is linked to resource acquisition and achievement. It triggers positive emotions such as joy, fun, and pleasure and is linked to activation of the mesolimbic reward system and dopamine production. It can also generate stress when linked to dominance-seeking and social positioning, which is associated with sympathetic nervous system activation and adrenaline production.

- The affiliative system provides information on personal safety and leads to experiences of warmth, kindness, acceptance, encouragement, support, and affiliation, as well as giving and receiving affection and care from others. It is linked to activation of the parasympathetic nervous system and production of oxytocin, endorphins, and other opioids.
- Many individuals oscillate between the threat and drive systems, with the affiliative system blocked or underutilized, which can lead to mental health problems. To create a healthy balance, the development of skills to shift the mind toward the affiliative system and down-regulate the threat and drive systems are crucial.
- From the standpoint of attachment theory, compassion is associated with the caregiving behavioural system—an innate system in parents and other caregivers to provide care for young children. This behavioural system is believed to have evolved mainly to complement the attachment behavioural system, which mediates individuals' emotional attachments to their caregivers.
- There are four different attachment styles in adults based on their early relationships with caregivers: secure, anxious, avoidant-dismissive, and avoidant-fearful. People with secure attachment style are confident, less easily threatened, and more readily available to help others than are insecure people. Insecure individuals with anxious attachment style tend to fixate on their own unmet needs and are less likely to help, while those with avoidant-dismissive or avoidant-fearful styles detach themselves from others.
- There is an intricate interplay between the attachment and caregiving behavioural systems. Activation of the attachment system (e.g., threat) can impede the functioning of the caregiving system by directing attention and resources to one's own protection and needs. Only when a sense of safety is present or reinstated can a would-be caregiver provide support to others in need.
- Compassion is innate and evolves to enhance the preservation of the human species through the development of physiological and psychological systems to support affiliative, prosocial, and compassionate thoughts, emotions, and behaviours.

- Compassion not only benefits the recipients; it also benefits the caregivers, too. Indeed, giving help has been shown to be a stronger predictor of better psychophysical health than is receiving help from others.

References

1. Gilbert P. The origins and nature of compassion focused therapy. *Br J Clin Psychol.* 2014;53(1):6–41.
2. Barkow JH. *Darwin, Sex and Status: Biological Approaches to Mind and Culture.* Toronto, ON: University of Toronto Press; 1989.
3. Baumeister RF, Leary MR. The need to belong: Desire for interpersonal attachments as a fundamental human motivation. *Psychol Bull.* 1995;117(3):497–529.
4. Crosier BS, Webster GD, Dillon HD. Wired to connect: Evolutionary psychology and social networks. *Annu Rev Psychol.* 2012;16:230–239.
5. Eisenberg N. Empathy-related emotional responses, altruism, and their socialization. In: Davidson R, Harrington A, eds. *Visions of Compassion: Western Scientists and Tibetan Buddhists Examine Human Nature.* New York: Oxford University Press; 2002: 131–164.
6. Penner LA, Dovidio JF, Piliavin JA, Schroeder DA. Prosocial behavior: Multilevel perspectives. *Annu Rev Psychol.* 2005;56:365–392.
7. Warneken F, Tomasello M. The roots of human altruism. *Br J Psychol.* 2009;100(Pt 3):455–471.
8. Warneken F, Tomasello M. Altruistic helping in human infants and young chimpanzees. *Science.* 2006;311(5765):1301–1303.
9. Baumeister RF, Bratslavsky E, Finkenauer C, Vohs KD. Bad is stronger than good. *Rev Gen Psychol.* 2001;5:323–370.
10. Gilbert P. Varieties of submissive behaviour: Their evolution and role in depression. In: Sloman L, Gilbert P, eds. *Subordination and Defeat: An Evolutionary Approach to Mood Disorders.* Hillsdale, NJ: Lawrence Erlbaum; 2000:3–46.
11. Berridge KC, Robinson TE. What is the role of dopamine in reward: Hedonic impact, reward learning, or incentive salience? *Brain Res Rev.* 1998;28(3):309–369.
12. Brewer J. *The Craving Mind: From Cigarettes to Smartphones to Love: Why We Get Hooked and How We Can Break Bad Habits.* New Haven, CT: Yale University Press; 2017.
13. Taylor PJ, Gooding P, Wood AM, Tarrier N. The role of defeat and entrapment in depression, anxiety, and suicide. *Psychol Bull.* 2011;137(3):391–420.

14. Porges SW. The polyvagal perspective. *Biol Psychol.* 2007;74(2):116–143.
15. Sapolsky RM. *Why Zebras Don't Get Ulcers.* New York: St Martin's Press; 1994.
16. Gilbert P. *The Compassionate Mind.* London: Constable & Robinson; 2009.
17. Bowlby J. *Attachment and Loss: Vol. 1. Attachment* (2nd ed.). New York: Basic Books; 1982.
18. Ainsworth MD, Bell SM. Attachment, exploration, and separation: Illustrated by the behavior of one-year-olds in a strange situation. *Child Dev.* 1970;41(1):49–67.
19. Cassidy J, Shaver PR, eds. *Handbook of Attachment: Theory, Research, and Clinical Applications* (3rd ed.). New York: Guilford Press; 2016.
20. Ainsworth MDS. Attachment and other affectional bonds across the life cycle. In: Parkes CM, Stevenson-Hinde J, Marris P, eds. *Attachment Across the Life Cycle.* New York: Routledge; 1991:3–51.
21. Mikulincer M, Shaver PR. An attachment perspective on compassion and altruism. In: Gilbert P, ed. *Compassion: Concepts, Research and Applications.* Oxon, UK: Routledge, Taylor & Francis Group; 2017:187–202.
22. Mikulincer M, Gillath O, Shaver PR. Activation of the attachment system in adulthood: Threat-related primes increase the accessibility of mental representations of attachment figures. *J Pers Soc Psychol.* 2002;83(4):881–895.
23. Cassidy J, Kobak RR. Avoidance and its relationship with other defensive processes. In: Belsky J, Nezworski T, eds. *Clinical Implications of Attachment.* Hillsdale, NJ: Erlbaum; 1988:300–323.
24. Mikulincer M, Shaver PR. *Attachment in Adulthood: Structure, Dynamics, and Change* (2nd ed.). New York: Guilford Press; 2016.
25. Brennan KA, Clark CL, Shaver PR. Self-report measurement of adult romantic attachment: An integrative overview. In: Simpson JA, Rholes WS, eds. *Attachment Theory and Close Relationships.* New York: Guilford Press; 1998:46–76.
26. Fraley RC. Adult attachment theory and research. A brief overview. http://labs.psychology.illinois.edu/~rcfraley/attachment.htm. Published 2018.
27. Bartholomew K, Horowitz LM. Attachment styles among young adults: A test of a four-category model. *J Pers Soc Psychol.* 1991;61(2):226–244.
28. Collins NL, Guichard AC, Ford MB, Feeney BC. Responding to need in intimate relationships: Normative processes and individual differences. In: Mikulincer M, Goodman GS, eds. *Dynamics of Romantic Love: Attachment, Caregiving, and Sex.* New York: Guilford Press; 2006:149–189.
29. Shaver PR, Mikulincer M, Gross JT, Stern JA, Cassidy J. A lifespan perspective on attachment and care for others: Empathy, altruism, and prosocial behavior. In: Cassidy J, Shaver PR, eds. *Handbook of Attachment: Theory,*

Research, and Clinical Applications (3rd ed.). New York: Guilford Press; 2016:e878–e916.

30. Burke SE, Wang K, Dovidio JF. Witnessing disclosure of depression: Gender and attachment avoidance moderate interpersonal evaluations. *J Soc Clin Psychol.* 2014;33:536–559.

31. Joireman JA, Needham TL, Cummings AL. Relationships between dimensions of attachment and empathy. *N Am J Psychol.* 2002;4:63–80.

32. Westmaas JL, Silver RC. The role of attachment in responses to victims of life crises. *J Pers Soc Psychol.* 2001;80(3):425–438.

33. Feeney BC, Cassidy J, Ramos-Marcuse F. The generalization of attachment representations to new social situations: Predicting behavior during initial interactions with strangers. *J Pers Soc Psychol.* 2008;95(6):1481–1498.

34. Mikulincer M, Gillath O, Halevy V, Avihou N, Avidan S, Eshkoli N. Attachment theory and reactions to others' needs: Evidence that activation of the sense of attachment security promotes empathic responses. *J Pers Soc Psychol.* 2001;81(6):1205–1224.

35. Mikulincer M, Gillath O, Sapir-Lavid Y, et al. Attachment theory and concern for others' welfare: Evidence that activation of the sense of secure base promotes endorsement of self-transcendence values. *Basic Appl Soc Psychol.* 2003;25:299–312.

36. Tosone C, Bettmann JE, Minami T, Jasperson RA. New York City social workers after 9/11: Their attachment, resiliency, and compassion fatigue. *Int J Emerg Ment Health.* 2010;12(2):103–116.

37. Pardess E, Mikulincer M, Dekel R, Shaver PR. Dispositional attachment orientations, contextual variations in attachment security, and compassion fatigue among volunteers working with traumatized individuals. *J Pers.* 2014;82(5):355–366.

38. Romaniello C, Farinelli M, Matera N, Bertoletti E, Pedone V, Northoff G. Anxious attachment style and hopelessness as predictors of burden in caregivers of patients with disorders of consciousness: A pilot study. *Brain Inj.* 2015;29(4):466–472.

39. Gilbert P, Irons C. Focused therapies and compassionate mind training for shame and self-attacking. In: Gilbert P, ed. *Compassion: Conceptualisations, Research and Use in Psychotherapy.* New York: Routledge; 2005:263–325.

40. Oman D, Thoresen CE. Spiritual modeling: A key to spiritual and religious growth? *Int J Psychol Relig.* 2003;13:149–165.

41. Yinon Y, Landau MO. On the reinforcing value of helping behavior in a positive mood. *Motiv Emot.* 1987;11:83–93.

42. Cialdini RB, Brown SL, Lewis BP, Luce C, Neuberg SL. Reinterpreting the empathy–altruism relationship: When one into one equals oneness. *J Pers Soc Psychol.* 1997;73:481–494.

43. Brunstein JC, Dangelmayer G, Schultheiss OC. Personal goals and social support in close relationships: Effects on relationship mood and marital satisfaction. *J Pers Soc Psychol.* 1996;71:1006–1019.

44. Schwartz C, Meisenhelder JB, Ma Y, Reed G. Altruistic social interest behaviors are associated with better mental health. *Psychosom Med.* 2003;65:778–785.

45. Brown SL, Nesse RM, Vinokur AD, Smith DM. Providing social support may be more beneficial than receiving it: Results from a prospective study of mortality. *Psychol Sci.* 2003;14:320–327.

46. Avlund K, Damsgaard MT, Holstein BE. Social relations and mortality: An eleven year follow-up study of 70-year-old men and women in Denmark. *Soc Sci Med.* 1998;47:635–643.

47. Brown WM, Consedine NS, Magai C. Altruism relates to health in an ethnically diverse sample of older adults. *J Gerontol B Psychol Sci Soc Sci.* 2005;60:143–152.

48. Hays J, Saunders W, Flint E, Kaplan B, Blazer DG. Social support and depression as risk factors for loss of physical function in late life. *Aging Ment Health.* 1997;1:209–220.

49. Brown SL, Brown RM, House JS, Smith DM. Coping with spousal loss: Potential buffering effects of self-reported helping behavior. *Pers Soc Psychol Bull.* 2008;34:849–861.

50. Roth DL, Haley WE, Hovater M, Perkins M, Wadley VG, Judd S. Family caregiving and all-cause mortality: Findings from a population-based propensity-matched analysis. *Am J Epidemiol.* 2013;178(10):1571–1578.

51. Brown SL, Smith DM, Schulz R, et al. Caregiving behavior is associated with decreased mortality risk. *Psychol Sci.* 2009;20:488–494.

52. Okun MA, Yeung EW, Brown S. Volunteering by older adults and risk of mortality: A meta-analysis. *Psychol Aging.* 2013;28(2):564–577.

53. Jenkinson CE, Dickens AP, Jones K, et al. Is volunteering a public health intervention? A systematic review and meta-analysis of the health and survival of volunteers. *BMC Public Health.* 2013;13:773.

54. Lum TY, Lightfoot E. The effects of volunteering on the physical and mental health of older people. *Res Aging.* 2005;27:31–55.

55. Brown RM, Brown SL. Informal caregiving: A reappraisal of effects on caregivers. *Soc Issues Policy Rev.* 2014;8:74–102.

56. Roth DL, Fredman L, Haley WE. Informal caregiving and its impact on health: A reappraisal from population-based studies. *Gerontologist.* 2015;55(2):309–319.

57. Poulin MJ, Brown SL, Ubel PA, Smith DM, Jankovic A, Langa KM. Does a helping hand mean a heavy heart? Helping behavior and well-being among spouse caregivers. *Psychol Aging.* 2010;25(1):108–117.

58. O'Reilly D, Connolly S, Rosato M, Patterson C. Is caring associated with an increased risk of mortality? A longitudinal study. *Soc Sci Med.* 2008;67(8):1282–1290.
59. Fredman L, Cauley JA, Hochberg M, Ensrud KE, Doros G. Mortality Associated with Caregiving, General Stress, and Caregiving-Related Stress in Elderly Women: Results of Caregiver-Study of Osteoporotic Fractures. *J Am Geriatr Soc.* 2010;58(5):937–943.
60. Figley CR. Introduction. In: Figley CR, ed. *Compassion Fatigue: Secondary Traumatic Stress Disorders from Treating the Traumatized.* New York: Brunner Mazel; 1995:xiii–xxii.
61. Figley CR, Figley KR. Compassion fatigue resilience. In: Seppälä EM, Simon-Thomas E, Brown SL, Worline MC, Cameron CD, Doty J, eds. *The Oxford Handbook of Compassion Science.* New York: Oxford University Press; 2017:387–398.

4

Is Compassion Innate? Spiritual and Eastern Perspectives

An Overview of Spiritual Perspectives

All faith traditions, worldwide, maintain that compassion underlies true spirituality and is a doorway to a transcendental relationship with what is variously called the Dao, God, Yahweh, Allah, Nirvana, or Brahman. From about 900–200 BCE, during what the German psychiatrist and philosopher Karl Jaspers coined the "Axial Age," a major shift (i.e., a turn, as if on an axis) occurred in which great intellectual, philosophical, and religious systems flourished and shaped the subsequent spiritual development of humanity.[1] In four different regions in the world, sages, prophets, mystics, logicians, and philosophers emerged: Confucianism and Daoism in ancient China; Hinduism, Buddhism, and Jainism on the Indian subcontinent; monotheism in the Middle East (which later gave rise to Rabbinic Judaism, Christianity, and Islam); and philosophical rationalism in ancient Greece.[1] These Axial Age originators displayed great ingenuity and yet, surprisingly, they all came to the same conclusion with respect to the universality of compassion, asserting that it is possible to reorient the mind from its self-centered, survivalistic, and potentially destructive instincts to focus on the welfare of others.

According to Karen Armstrong, a renowned comparative religion scholar, although each faith tradition expresses it differently, compassion can be summed up aptly by the Golden Rule: "Do unto others as you would have them do unto you," "which asks us to look into our own hearts, discover what gives us pain, and then refuse, under any circumstance whatsoever, to inflict that pain on anybody else."[2] For example, in the Analects (15.23), Confucius said: "[O]ne word sums up the basis of all good conduct . . . loving-kindness. Do not do to others what you do not want done to yourself," whereas in Hinduism, a similar maxim appeared: "[T]his is the sum of duty: do not do to others what would cause pain if done to you" (Mahabharata 5:1517). The three major monotheistic religions would also agree. Hillel, one of the most influential rabbis in Rabbinic Judaism, said: "What is hateful to you, do not do to your neighbour. This is the whole Torah; all the rest is commentary" (Shabbat 31a). In Christianity, Jesus said: "In everything, do to others as you would have them do to you; for this is the law and the prophets" (Matthew 7:12). Finally, in Islam, the Prophet Muhammad said: "Not one of you truly believes until you wish for others what you wish for yourself" (Hadith). Indeed, in Semitic languages, the word for compassion (*rahamim* in biblical Hebrew, *rahamanut* in post-biblical Hebrew, and *rahman* in Arabic) is related etymologically to *rehem* or womb, denoting motherly or sibling (coming from the same womb), love that gives rise to unselfish, unconditional regard for others.

The Golden Rule alerts us to our everyday self-absorption and reminds us that we are equal to others who deserve the same consideration we give to ourselves. It asks us to transcend our ego by cutting through our habitual preoccupation that narrowly focuses on survival, material gain, and achievement. It teaches us that shedding our ego—by refraining from doing harm, performing good deeds, and being compassionate to others—is indispensable to transcendence. For example, the Chinese Daoist philosopher and mystic Zhuangzi said, "The perfect man has no self," a characteristic that is essential for the "great transformation" of the Way or *Dao*.[3] Buddhists also teach about "no-self" (*anattā*), a key to attaining sublime peace. Similarly, early Christians spoke of a new freedom in which God "exalted him to the highest place" (Philippians 2:6–11) when they, like Jesus, emptied themselves of egotism.[2] The rabbis also maintained that when a Jew studied the Torah for its own sake rather than for personal gain, he became "the Beloved Companion. . . . And it makes him great and lifts him above the entire creation."[4] The relationship between "non-self," compassion, and transcendence is summed up elegantly by one of the greatest minds of the 20th century, Nobel laureate Albert Einstein, who wrote:

A human being is a part of the whole, called by us "Universe," a part limited in time and space. He experiences himself, his thoughts and feeling as something separated from the rest, a kind of optical delusion of his consciousness. This delusion is a kind of prison for us, restricting us to our personal desires and to affection for a few persons nearest to us. Our task must be to free ourselves from this prison by widening our circle of compassion to embrace all living creatures and the whole of nature in its beauty. Nobody is able to achieve this completely but striving for such achievement is, in itself, a part of the liberation and a foundation for inner security.[5]

As we can see, compassion is universal among all major religions as well as among people with no religious faith. Indeed, the Charter of Compassion, composed by six faith traditions (Judaism, Christianity, Islam, Hinduism, Buddhism, and Confucianism) and launched in 2009, affirms that

the principle of compassion lies at the heart of all religious, ethical, and spiritual traditions, calling us always to treat all others as we wish to be treated ourselves. Compassion impels us to work tirelessly to alleviate the suffering of our fellow creatures, to dethrone ourselves from the centre of our world and put another there, and to honour the inviolable sanctity of every single human being, treating everybody, without exception, with absolute justice, equity, and respect.[2]

Since its inception, the Charter has been signed by more than 2 million people from around the world, and it has partnered with hundreds of interfaith organizations and cities.[6] It has been enshrined in synagogues, mosques, temples, and churches, as well as in secular institutions such as the Sydney Opera House and Karachi Press Club.[2]

As we can see, each of the world spiritual traditions has its own particular insight into the nature of compassion, and each has something unique to offer. When we investigate and reflect on the teachings on compassion from our own tradition, it would be valuable to open ourselves to explore other traditions as well. By doing so, we can begin to appreciate what other human beings hold in common, no matter their origin, culture, or beliefs. Through this process, we can enrich our own understanding of the tradition to which we belong.

In the next section, I dive deeper into the Eastern perspectives on compassion, with special attention given to the Buddhist view partly because of my personal interests and experience, but mostly because many contemporary secular compassion training programs borrow the mind-training tools that originate with Buddhism. This exploration also sets an important stage for the next chapter, in which I combine Western scientific evidence and Eastern ancient teachings to address whether compassion is trainable from a neuroscientific perspective.

Confucianism and the Golden Rule

The first known person to set forth the Golden Rule was the Chinese sage Confucius (孔子; 551–479 BCE), who made it the foundation of his philosophy. He called the rule or principle *zhong-shu* (忠恕), which can be summarized by the maxim "never do to others what you would not like them do to you (己所不欲,勿施於人)."[7] "*Shu*" means consideration or likening to oneself, and Confucius explicitly depicted it as human-heartedness, akin to compassion.[8] In the West, Confucius is often seen as a ritualist, obsessed with the minutiae of rules or *li* (禮). However, his underlying motivation to revive ancient rites was to control egotism and cultivate compassion during the "Spring and Autumn Period" (春秋時代) when small kingdoms attempted to defeat one another with barbaric cruelty, deceits, and impunity. The rituals of consideration (*shu*) ensured that people did not treat others based on self-interest but out of a sacred respect for every human being and the virtue of "yielding" to their fellows.[2] Thus, the principle of consideration is based on an egalitarian notion that recognizes the equal worth of all beings and that takes the particular characteristics and desires of others into consideration. Later scholars emphasized that Confucius' Golden Rule requires a dual practice: acquiring firsthand observation through personal experience (*zhong*) and imagining oneself in the position of the other (*shu*).[9] According to Confucius, by practising the Golden Rule "all day and every day," a person would become a "mature human being" or *junzi* (君子) and achieve the ideal noble quality of humanity or *ren* (仁).[7] Thus, compassion is inseparable from humanity, and the diligent practice of the Golden Rule removes us from our egocentricity, leading us to a spiritual awakening of the Way or *Dao* (道).

Daoism and the Way

Laozi (老子; 6th–4th century BCE) and Zhuangzi (莊子; 370–311 BCE) are pivotal figures in classical philosophical Daoism and are the chief sages of the Axial Age. They sought to live a life that is in harmony with the Way (*Dao*)—the origin of the sky and earth, the mother of all myriad things, and the potential that makes nature the way it is.[10] Yet while nature is in constant flux, we tend to think that things are permanent, believing mistakenly that what we perceive is all of reality. These sages taught us that it is our ego that makes us identify with our opinions, disagree with others, and harm one another. They asked us to return to a deep inner stillness, and just like "muddy water that becomes clear on its own when not agitated,"[10] we can begin to see the constantly changing nature of all myriad things. When we begin to appreciate the insubstantiality of all things, including the self, we naturally let go of our self-importance and, from there, forbearance, magnanimity, and benevolence that exclude nothing emerge. Without the distorting lens of self-centredness, "emptiness" reflects other things and people "like a mirror." This leads spontaneously to compassion for all, such that when "people cry, so he cries—he considers everything as his own being."[3] From this all-inclusive stance comes a "kingliness of character" that is "heaven-like," and a person with such character is said to possess the Way.[10]

Buddhist Perspective on Compassion

Like Confucius, the Buddha (470–390 BCE) also emphasized the importance of firsthand observation through personal experience and the inseparability of compassion in all beings. In fact, the aspiration to awakening (*bodhicitta*; 菩提心) is said to arise from both compassion (*karuṇā*; 悲)[*] and wisdom (*prajña*; *paññā*; 般若) in order to help others awaken to life. This is illustrated by the Four Noble Truths, the first and foremost teaching that the Buddha gave upon his enlightenment.[11] The first truth—the truth of suffering (*duḥkha*; *dukkha*; 苦)—asks us to look deeply into our own suffering. As we do, we begin to see the suffering of others, we gradually develop a deep insight into the impersonal and universal nature of suffering; that is, *the* suffering, rather than *my* or *their* suffering. The second truth—the cause of suffering—points out that suffering arises from attachment (when we don't get what we want), aversion (when we get what we don't want), and ignorance (when we mistakenly believe that things are permanent and that we are separate from others). The third truth—cessation of suffering—pronounces that there is a realm of transcendental peace within each person called *nirvāṇa* (*nibbana*; 涅槃) wherein all causes of suffering are "extinguished like a flame." The fourth truth—the path to the cessation of suffering—asserts that there is a path that we can follow to attain *nirvāṇa* through the cultivation of morality, meditation, and wisdom.[11,12] Thus, we can see a compassionate arc in the Four Noble Truths: transcendental peace (third truth) can be reached by first touching deeply into our own suffering (first truth) to understand its universal nature and its cause (second truth). This understanding leads to the motivation to follow the path (fourth truth) so that all beings, including oneself, can be liberated from suffering to realize a state of genuine well-being.

The early Buddhist view on compassion is the wish for others to be relieved from suffering. It holds that the *act of seeing* the actual suffering of others does not qualify as compassion, although realizing others' suffering is often a pre-condition for compassion to arise. It cautions that in mentally dwelling on the suffering of others, the object of contemplation by the practitioner is *suffering*—which can generate grief or sadness. In contrast, in the cultivation of compassion,

---

[*] For special terms, I have used Sanskrit words in the first instance of appearance because Sanskrit is the language conventionally used in the academic discipline of Buddhist Studies. The Sanskrit words are accompanied by their cognate forms in Pāli (if available) and traditional Chinese characters in parenthesis.

the object of contemplation is *freedom from suffering*—which can generate a positive or even joyful mind. Understood in this way, from a Buddhist perspective, compassion does not mean to commiserate with others' suffering, which elicits personal suffering; rather, it represents a positive, often joyful state of active motivation for others to be free from suffering and affliction. This distinction has influenced and is congruent with the modern Western understanding of compassion (feeling *with* other's suffering) versus empathy (feeling *into* other's suffering); the latter, when unregulated, could lead to personal or empathic distress.[13]

The foundation for compassionate activity is the meditative practice of compassion. Meditation on compassion strengthens the compassionate disposition of one's own mind, so that one could ideally respond spontaneously and skilfully when a situation that calls for compassion arises. Interestingly, unlike its contemporary counterpart, compassion as a meditation practice in the early Buddhist notion takes the form of a boundless radiation in all directions that lacks any reference to an object or specific being. This early focus on boundless radiation is in contradistinction to later instructions, which explicitly take actual persons—such as a friend, a neutral person, and an enemy—in turn as the objects of meditation and gradually expand one's practice until it becomes boundless and universal. These later instructions can be viewed as a skilful approach in the initial stages of meditation practice when one's stability is not strong enough, so that one can gradually develop more meditative skills to eventually take the form of boundless radiation.

The concept of compassion underwent great changes around the 4th century CE, with the development of the bodhisattva (*bodhisattva*; 菩薩) ideal. Bodhisattvas are awakened beings, who, seeing the pervasiveness of sufferings, aspire and take vows to go through numerous cycles of self-sacrifice to seek ultimate wisdom.[14] For these awakened beings, the motive of "great compassion" to save all beings from suffering becomes their *raison d'être* to pursue intellectual understanding; to learn secular subjects such as mathematics, medicine, and the arts; and to study the scriptures, as well as to meditate in order to penetrate further into the ultimate truth. Thus, in later traditions, there is a strong emphasis that the pursuit of ultimate wisdom should be motivated for the welfare of all beings, rather than one's own liberation only. Indeed, the importance of developing both wisdom and compassion has been compared to two wings of a bird: serving others without a deep source of wisdom leads to harm and exhaustion, whereas pursuing wisdom without deep compassion leads to a disengaged, self-centered aloofness.[12] This interdependent relationship has been epitomized aptly in the adage: "Wisdom without compassion is bondage. Compassion without wisdom is bondage."[12]

The Four Immeasurables

For more than 2,500 years, the cultivation of compassion has been practised traditionally alongside loving-kindness, sympathetic joy, and equanimity. Together, they are known as the four *brahmavihāras* (梵住), the four divine abodes, or the four immeasurables (*appamāṇa*; *appammaññā*; 無量心), and their order is important (see later discussion).[15] Like compassion, the other three immeasurables are also characterized by boundlessness, a spacious mind-state that radiates in all directions and indiscriminately.[15]

The practices of the four immeasurables predated the historical Buddha and were commonly discussed among members of Vedic or orthodox Brahmanical traditions in ancient India and their contemporaries.[15] For example, three of the four immeasurables— loving-kindness, compassion, and equanimity—could be found in the later Upanishads, the sacred treatises of Hinduism.[16] In Jainism literature, similar components also could be found with some slight variations—loving-kindness, compassion, delight/satisfaction (*prāmodya*, which is a cognate of *muditā* or sympathetic joy), and nonattachment.[16]

In what follows, I will explore the four immeasurables, their similarities and differences, as well as the relationships among them. This will allow us to better appreciate the Eastern views on compassion. In addition, an understanding of the overlapping conceptual and psychological components of the four immeasurables may illuminate distinctions in the underlying neural networks during their deliberate training, a topic that I will review in the next chapter.

Loving-Kindness (maitrī; mettā; 慈*).* Loving-kindness, or benevolence, is the first and the most frequently mentioned immeasurable in the early discourses. The etymological root of *maitrī* is *mitra,* or "friend," which conveys an attitude of friendliness and cordiality in interpersonal relationships, as well as a general wish for another's welfare, irrespective of external conditions or personal circumstances. Loving-kindness plays a foundational role for the cultivation of the other three immeasurables and has been described as the "water" that nourishes the roots of the tree of compassion.[15] Loving-kindness is directly opposed to hostility or ill will (*vyāpāda;* 瞋), its far enemy (Box 4.1). Indeed, the cultivation of loving-kindness deprives ill will of its nourishment.[15] Therefore, loving-kindness is the antidote to anger, ill will, and aggression when these mental states arise within oneself or when one is facing others who act under their grip.[15,17] Selfish attachment is the near enemy (a subtle mental state that is blemished by a sense of self-concern or indifference), which, similar to loving-kindness, is characterized by affection toward another being, but, unlike loving-kindness, it is stained by an unwholesome craving (*tṛṣṇā;* 愛), or self-centered wanting, that results from dissatisfaction and a perceived sense of lack.[18] By comparing it to its enemies, loving-kindness can be described as a benevolence that is devoid of

---

Box 4.1 The Near and Far Enemies of the Four Immeasurables.[15,17,19,20]

Immeasurables	English translation	Near enemy	Far enemy
Maitrī	Loving-kindness, benevolence	Selfish attachment, greed	Hostility, ill will
Karuṇā	Compassion	Grief, sadness, pity	Cruelty
Muditā	Sympathetic joy	Frivolous joy	Envy, jealousy, *schadenfreude*
Upekṣā	Equanimity, equipoise	Apathy, indifference	Agitation

selfish concern, a state that is essential to establishing cordiality in relation to others and that diminishes the proclivity to hostility, ill will, and anger.

Compassion (*karuṇā* and *anukampā*). The second immeasurable is compassion. It has three forms: referential, insight-based, and nonreferential.[21–23] The first form, what social psychologists call "referential compassion," is familiar to most of us. It is a kind of compassion that we give to those we care about and have strong connections with—our children, partners, parents, friends, pets, neighbours, and fellows of the same ethnic or cultural group—in essence, our in-group. It can be directed to those we are not familiar with, such as the homeless, refugees, and victims of natural disasters, abuses, and violence. It can also flow to animals, plants, and the earth. From a Buddhist perspective, referential compassion is based on the view that sentient beings actually *exist*. It is what the *Vimalakīrtinirdeśa Sutra* (*Vimalakīrti's Instructions*; 維摩經) refers to as "sentimental compassion" because it is marked by affection toward those with whom we share close connections or similar experiences and by false views that are based on distinction between self and others.

While referential compassion is highly valued in our culture, most of us are less acquainted with the other forms of compassion. Insight-based compassion, the second form, is more conceptual. Roshi Joan Halifax, a Buddhist teacher and Zen priest who founded the Upaya Institute and Zen Center, in her book *Standing at the Edge*, writes about this kind of compassion as a moral imperative—the "right" thing to do in face of suffering and an affirmation of respect and dignity—because we can "deduce that ignoring suffering can have serious consequences for self, other, and society."[20] The concept of insight-based compassion, which also exists in Tibetan Buddhism, is based on impermanence, non-self, and interdependence/interconnectedness. It comes from the realization that the boundaries between the lives of all beings are true only in the conventional sense because, in reality, there is actually no separateness of distinct lives. It arises from seeing clearly the illusory nature of all existence, sentient and nonsentient.

The third form, nonreferential (objectless) compassion, is unbiased, boundless, and universal. It is a compassion without object, what the Zen master Soseki called "true compassion."[21–23] Roshi Joan Halifax, quoting the late Roshi Hakuun Yasutani, writes that nonreferential compassion is when "the compassion of the undifferentiated body of no-cause comes burning forth." It is the essence of Avalokiteśvara (a bodhisattva who embodies compassion) who hears the cries of the world "with a boundless heart—one that does not sink like a heavy stone in the waters of suffering but is broken open like a geode to the rare space within, glittering with light for those who are struggling in darkness."[20] Nonreferential compassion is based on the realization of boundlessness/emptiness—nothing has objective, independent, ultimate existence. It is manifested in someone who has a deep, whole-hearted practice, or who is naturally predisposed, as in enlightened beings, Buddhas, Tantric *siddhas* (adepts), and other advanced bodhisattvas.

The spirit of nonreferential compassion is vividly illustrated by a story of Asaṅga, a 4th-century master. Asaṅga went into retreat for 12 years to cultivate compassion and meditate on Maitreya, the Buddha of loving-kindness. He was somewhat disappointed when he did not receive any vision from Maitreya. After finishing the retreat, he met a miserable red dog with a rotting wound in its hindquarters. Seeing that the wound was infested by maggots, Asaṅga wanted to remove them, but realized that they needed flesh to stay alive. So, he cut a slice of flesh from his own leg to feed them. In order not to cause any harm to the maggots, he then used his own tongue to lick them off the dog. At that very moment, the red dog transformed into Maitreya and told Asaṅga that he had been with Asaṅga all along, but could not be seen until Asaṅga took action to serve another being. From this story, we can see that nonreferential compassion is brought forth by a heart and mind that are open to the suffering of all sentient beings—like the moon casting its reflection indiscriminately on a hundred bowls of water—and one that is ready to serve in an instant.[20]

According to the *Vimalakīrti's Instructions*, referential compassion "exhausts the bodhisattva" and therefore must be transcended into insight-based and nonreferential compassion, which do not exhaust the practitioner. For this reason, those who possess nonreferential compassion can accomplish unlimited bodhisattva deeds for the welfare of all beings. In this regard, the emphasis of ancient Buddhist teaching on the progressive development of the three types of compassion is highly relevant in the contemporary world, especially for healthcare professionals who are susceptible to burnout, cynicism, and empathic distress.

The far enemy of compassion is cruelty, a mental state that is directly opposed to compassion and leads to future suffering. Easily masquerading as compassion, grief,[17] sadness,[15] or pity[24] are its near enemies, because they share in their confrontation with the suffering of others, but are different in that they evoke personal suffering.

Sympathetic Joy (*muditā*; 喜). The third immeasurable is sympathetic joy. Etymologically, *muditā*, is closely related to the words *prāmodya* (*pāmojja*), or delight, and *anumodana* (*anumodana*; 隨喜), or rejoicing. It is characterized by rejoicing in the successes of others[15] and is described as being brought about naturally when one lives harmoniously with others in a context of mutual appreciation and concern for their well-being. Sympathetic joy leads, via tranquility and happiness, to concentration, a key to meditative practice. As a positive emotion elicited by that of others, sympathetic joy could be considered as a type of empathy since it requires feeling into another's mental and affective states. Sympathetic joy has two far enemies. The first far enemy is envy, a feeling of discontented or resentful longing aroused by someone else's successes, possessions, qualities, or luck. The second far enemy is *schadenfreude*, pleasure that is derived from others' misfortunes. Sympathetic joy also eradicates personal discontent (*arāti*; *arati*).[15] The near enemy of sympathetic joy is frivolous joy,[19] a type of joy that arises from an egoistic, compulsive search for pleasures that is driven by craving to find temporary relief from underlying dissatisfaction. Similar to the other immeasurables, sympathetic joy represents a positive, tranquil state that arises from the welfare of others, rather than a pleasure that arises from self-focused craving.

Equanimity (*upekṣā*; *upekkhā*; 捨). The fourth immeasurable is equanimity, or equipoise. Etymologically, *upekṣā* suggests a mental attitude of "looking upon" and not an indifferent "looking away." Equanimity conveys an awareness of whatever is happening combined with a sense of mental equilibrium and the absence of favouring or opposing, one that "rounds off a systematic opening of the heart."[18] There are two main usages of the term "equanimity." The first refers to a neutral feeling (*vedanā*; 受), a mental state that is neither pleasant nor unpleasant. It involves neither "intensifying nor dampening current mental states"[25] and is experienced commonly during ordinary life. This first usage corresponds to the Western psychological notion of "neutral valence."[26] The second usage of equanimity corresponds to a nonpreferential mind. It is an "even-mindedness in the face of every sort of experience, regardless of whether pleasure or pain are present or not"[27] and "a state of mind that cannot be swayed by biases and preferences."[25] This state of equanimity manifests as "a balanced reaction to joy and misery, which protects one from emotional agitation."[28] In this second usage, equanimity is very similar to the psychological constructs of "decentring" and "nonattachment"—mechanisms that help one to disengage from one's thoughts and emotions.[29] The far enemy of equanimity is agitated reactivity, a disturbed mental state in which one is dissatisfied because external circumstances do not match one's personal expectation or preference. Apathy, a dull indifference or neutrality toward experience is the near enemy of equanimity.[19]

The Four Immeasurables in Context. A common thread that runs through the four immeasurables is the emptying of self-concern,[15] which can be seen by examining their far and near enemies. The far enemies depict negative mental states and harmful intentions directed to others, whereas the near enemies, though seemingly positive on the surface, represent mental states that are blemished by a sense of self-concern or indifference. Far and near enemies are in contrast to the four immeasurables, which distinctively represent positive, other-oriented emotional responses that are devoid of self-centred desires and cravings. It is from this selfless state that one deliberately cultivates prosocial intentions and the ability to feel positively *for* others, irrespective of others' emotional state (suffering, joy, etc.) or whether there is a concrete target.

Compassion and Its Relationship to the Other Immeasurables. The basic thrust of compassion is the wish to alleviate the suffering of others. A potential pitfall of compassion could arise when one habitually perceives others as less fortunate or being in an inferior position, leading one to develop a sense of superiority or conceit. One way to counterbalance this possible pitfall is to contextualize compassion by cultivating it together with the other immeasurables.[15] Here, the foundational building can be done by way of loving-kindness, which takes its objects indiscriminately and impartially—whether the objects are better or worse, lovable or unlovable. The cultivation of loving-kindness thus complements that of compassion by deliberately training one to develop the ability to treat everyone equally as one's friend, thereby counteracting the dualistic sense of superiority and inferiority. The cultivation of compassion that is primarily concerned with those in a less favourable situation also has its natural complement in sympathetic joy, which allows those in a more favourable situation to be integrated into one's four immeasurables practice. The cultivation of sympathetic joy thus ensures that what is positive also receives due attention.

With equanimity, a further complement comes into play. While loving-kindness, compassion, and sympathetic joy each has a direct relationship to others, equanimity complements these three immeasurables as a selfless and impartial joy that arises without an active target.[15] While equanimity is not the most skilful response in many situations, in others, it clearly is the appropriate response. When compassionate activity meets an unreceptive response (e.g., a difficult patient who defies all medical recommendations repeatedly), then perhaps the time has come to give up attempts to control the situation or change it for the better and move on to equanimity. This requires one to allow others to take responsibility for their own actions and attitudes. In this way, equanimity "rounds off" the cultivation of compassion by "freeing it from any trace of compulsion and obsession."[15] The presence of equanimity makes the set of the four immeasurables complete. The four immeasurables, thus, as a whole, offer the practitioner a complete range of choices for the cultivation of appropriate mental attitudes in any kind of situation.

Self-Compassion and Western Psychology

The concept of self-compassion has garnered much attention in recent years.[30] It is based on the notion of the self in Western psychology— a "definable knowable entity with particular characteristics, universal needs, and somewhat predictable developmental thrusts."[31] Buddhism, on the other hand, takes a radically different approach toward the potential of the self and its relationship to reality, with im-permanence, non-self, and non-duality being its central tenets.

Self-compassion originates from loving-kindness meditation in Buddhism, which directs practitioners to extend compassion to-ward all living beings, including oneself.[32] It is comprised of three components: mindfulness, common humanity, and self-kindness.[33] While mindfulness is at the heart of Buddhist teachings, the two other components of self-compassion—common humanity and self-kindness—do not accord entirely with the classic Buddhist world-view. Why? Although common humanity highlights the shared connections among human beings, the underlying philosophy is that of separation of self from others, which differs from the emphasis on non-self and non-duality in Buddhist philosophy.[34] In addition, self-kindness focuses on the happiness of oneself, whereas Buddhism stresses the deliberate co-cultivation of the four immeasurables for the benefits of all beings. As a new development from Western psy-chology, self-compassion could be considered a form of self-care and what social psychologists called "referential compassion." Without dwelling further on the difference between this Western psycho-logical construct and the conservative Buddhist viewpoint, to avoid confusion or further controversy, I will use the term "inner com-passion"—the ability to turn understanding, acceptance and love inward toward self, especially when dealing with self-criticism—in the remainder of this book. From a practical standpoint, it should be emphasized that the active cultivation of inner compassion is a pow-erful antidote to burnout, especially in healthcare, a topic that I will discuss in Chapter 7.

Summary of Key Points

- Although each faith tradition expresses it differently, compassion can be summed up aptly by the Golden Rule: "Do unto others as you would have them do unto you." The Charter of Compassion affirms that "the principle of compassion lies at the heart of all re-ligious, ethical, and spiritual traditions, calling us always to treat all others as we wish to be treated ourselves."

- From a Buddhist perspective, compassion does not mean to commiserate with others' suffering. Rather, it represents a positive, often joyful state of active motivation for others to be free from suffering and affliction.
- "Wisdom without compassion is bondage. Compassion without wisdom is bondage"—serving others without a deep source of wisdom leads to harm and exhaustion, whereas pursuing wisdom without deep compassion leads to a disengaged, self-centered aloofness.
- The meditative cultivation of compassion has been practised traditionally alongside loving-kindness, sympathetic joy, and equanimity. Together, they are called the four immeasurables.
- Loving-kindness is the wish for others to be happy. Its far enemy is hostility or ill will, whereas its near enemy is attachment or greed.
- There are three forms compassion: referential, insight-based, and nonreferential. Referential compassion is marked by affection toward those we care about. Insight-based compassion is based on the knowledge that we are interdependent and the insight that ignoring suffering can have serious consequences for self, other, and society. Nonreferential compassion is unbiased, boundless, universal, and without object. The far enemy of compassion is cruelty, whereas its near enemies are grief, sadness, and pity.
- Sympathetic joy is rejoicing in the successes of others. Its far enemies are envy, jealousy, and *schadenfreude*, whereas its near enemy is frivolous joy.
- Equanimity is a sense of mental equilibrium, the absence of favouring or opposing, and seeing things as they are. It corresponds to the Western psychological notions of neutral valence, decentring, and nonattachment. Its far enemy is agitation, whereas its near enemy is apathy or indifference.

References

1. Jaspers K. *The Origin and Goal of History.* Oxon, UK: Routledge; 2010.
2. Armstrong K. *Twelve Steps to a Compassionate Life.* New York: Alfred A. Knopf; 2010.

3. Palmer M, Breuilly E, Chang WM, Ramsay J. *The Book of Chuang Tzu.* London: Penguin Books; 2006.
4. Fishbane MA. *The Garments of Torah: Essays in Biblical Hermeneutics.* Bloomington: Indiana University Press; 1989.
5. Sullivan W. The Einstein papers. A man of many parts. *The New York Times*; Mar 29, 1972.
6. Charter for Compassion. https://charterforcompassion.org/.
7. Confucius. *The Analects.* New York: Penguin Classics; 1962.
8. Puka B. The Golden Rule. Internet encyclopedia of philosophy. A peer-reviewed academic resource. https://www.iep.utm.edu/goldrule/. Published 2020.
9. Wang C. Confucius' Zhong-Shu and Zhuangzi's Qiwu: Zhang Taiyan's parallel interpretation. *Dao.* 2017;16:53–71.
10. Roberts M. *Dao De Jing: The Book of the Way.* Berkeley: University of California Press; 2001.
11. Thich Nhat Hahn. *The Heart of the Buddha's Teaching: Transforming Suffering into Peace, Joy, and Liberation.* New York: Harmony Books; 2015.
12. Wallace BA. *Buddhism with an Attitude: The Tibetan Seven-Point Mind Training.* Ithaca, NY: Snow Lion Publications; 2003.
13. Singer T, Klimecki OM. Empathy and compassion. *Curr Biol.* 2014;24(18):R875–R878.
14. Dayal H. *The Bodhisattva Doctrine in Buddhist Sanskrit Literature.* Delhi: Motilal Banarsidas; 1970.
15. Anālayo Bhikkhu. *Compassion and Emptiness in Early Buddhist Meditation.* Cambridge: Windhorse Publications; 2015.
16. Wiltshire MG. *Ascetic Figures Before and in Early Buddhism: The Emergence of Gautama as the Buddha.* New York: Mouton de Gruyter; 1990.
17. Ñāṇamoli Bhikkhu. *The Path of Purification: Visuddhimagga.* Kandy, Sri Lanka: Buddhist Publication Society; 1991.
18. Anālayo Bhikkhu. *Excursions into the Thought-World of the Pāli Discourses.* Onalaska, WA: Pariyatti Publishing; 2012.
19. Jinpa T. *A Fearless Heart: How the Courage to Be Compassionate Can Transform Our Lives.* New York: Hudson Street Press; 2015.
20. Halifax J. *Standing at the Edge.* New York: Martin's Press; 2018.
21. Soseki M. *Dialogues in a Dream.* Somerville, MA: Wisdom Publications; 2015.
22. Thurman R. *The Holy Teaching of Vimalakīrti.* University Park: Pennsylvania State University Press; 2000.
23. Gómez L. Emptiness and moral perfection. *Philos East West.* 1973;23(3):361–372.
24. Kornfield J. *A Path with Heart: A Guide Through the Perils and Promises of Spiritual Life.* New York: Bantam Books; 1993.

25. Bodhi Bhikkhu. *A Comprehensive Manual of Abhidhamma: The Philosophical Psychology of Buddhism.* Onalaska, WA: Buddhist Publication Society; 2000.
26. Desbordes G, Gard T, Hoge EA, et al. Moving beyond mindfulness: Defining equanimity as an outcome measure in meditation and contemplative research. *Mindfulness.* 2015;6(2):356–372.
27. Thanissaro Bhikkhu. *The Wings to Awakening An Anthology from the Pali Canon.* Barre, MA: Dhamma Dana Publications; 1996.
28. Bodhi Bhikkhu. *In the Buddha's Words: An Anthology of Discourses from the Pali Canon.* Somerville, MA: Wisdom Publications; 2005.
29. Vago DR, Silbersweig DA. Self-awareness, self-regulation, and self-transcendence (S-ART): A framework for understanding the neurobiological mechanisms of mindfulness. *Front Hum Neurosci.* 2012;6:296.
30. Barnard LK, Curry JF. Self-compassion: Conceptualizations, correlates, & interventions. *Rev Gen Psychol* 2011;15(4):289–303.
31. Donner SE. Self or no self: Views from self psychology and Buddhism in a postmodern context. *Smith Coll Stud Soc Work.* 2010;80:215–227.
32. Neff K. Self-compassion: An alternative conceptualization of a healthy attitude toward oneself. *Self Identity.* 2003;2:85–101.
33. Neff KD. The development and validation of a scale to measure self-compassion. *Self Identity.* 2003;2:223–250.
34. Peng Y, Shen J. The analysis of self-compassion and self-construal in the compassion-contemplation of Buddhism. *Advances in Psychol Sci.* 2012;20:1479–1486.

5

East Meets West

Is Compassion Trainable? A Neuroscientific Perspective

While compassion is cherished among all major wisdom-based traditions, Buddhism has developed an extensive set of mind-training tools to cultivate compassion systematically through meditation, contemplation, and insights or wisdom. Indeed, these ancient techniques have formed the basis of many contemporary secular mindfulness and compassion training programs. What is most interesting is that these well-defined skills also lend themselves to "testable hypotheses" that have fuelled many scientific investigations in the past two decades. We now have accumulating evidence showing the many beneficial effects of cultivating mindfulness and compassion, and, importantly, both are trainable skills. In this chapter, I attempt an East–West synthesis of compassion from a neuroscience perspective. It should be noted that different Buddhist traditions have their own unique emphasises, goals, and approaches to the cultivation of compassion that have been adopted by different secular programs. I will use the term "training" in the remainder of this chapter, acknowledging that, as a student of Buddhism, I am bound to over-generalize and over-simplify the unfathomable and nuanced teachings that these diverse traditions have to offer.

Mindfulness: Attentional Foundations of Compassion Practice

Before I explore the neuroscience of compassion, a brief review of two foundational contemplative skills—focused attention (*śamatha; samatha; 止*) and open monitoring (*vipaśyanā; vipassana;*

觀)—and their neural pathways are in order, for two main reasons. First, the ability to minimize self-concerns and regulate other-oriented emotions, as demonstrated by the four immeasurables, are interrelated with and built upon proficiency in these two antecedent contemplative skills. Second, a review of these skills allows us to address a central question: What are the benefits and the neural mechanisms involved during the cultivation of compassion that are *above and beyond* those shared with mindfulness trainings?

The first of two distinct but interrelated attentional practices is called *focused attention*.[1] According to Buddhist practice, focused attention deliberately trains sustained attention and reduces mental distraction, and it belongs to a larger body of meditation practices that foster concentration (*samādhi*; 三昧), which means "to collect." It is often called "one-pointedness" meditation because it directs the mind to focus firmly and exclusively on a single point, such as the breath or an image, leading to serenity and mental calm.[2,3] For concentration to be sustained, one must recognize when distractions arise and skilfully redirect attention back to the focused object.[3-6] Thus, focused attention primarily reinforces the ability to maintain a stable, alert, and concentrated state on the one hand, and disengage and reorient attention back to a focused object on the other.[5]

The second practice is called *insight* or *open monitoring*. While focused attention focuses on a single object, open monitoring anchors the mind to the present while broadening it to encompass the whole flux of internal and external experiences as they arise and pass away from moment to moment. With practice, it leads to insights into the transient and insubstantial nature of all phenomena and experiences including thoughts, feelings, and bodily sensations. Open monitoring meditation is typically associated with cultivating mindfulness (*smṛti*; *satī*; 念).[7] The literal translation of *smṛti* is "to remember." Thus, mindfulness connotes both awareness and memory in the sense that, by anchoring attention to present moment experiences, memory is facilitated. Indeed, mindfulness has been shown to enhance both working and episodic memory.[8-10]

In what follows, I review the growing body of research showing that training in focused attention and open monitoring enhance attention through the modulation of attentional resources. Interestingly,

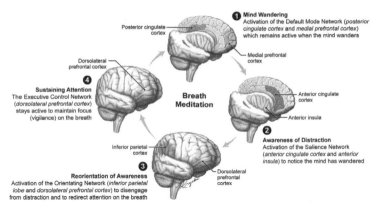

Figure 5.1 How the attention networks work together during mindfulness/focused attention meditation. Arousal and alertness are maintained by the alerting network (not shown). (1) When the mind wanders, the default mode network becomes activated. (2) The salience network (a subsystem of the executive control network) detects that the meditator has been distracted. (3) The orienting network disengages the meditator from distraction, redirecting attention back on the breath. (4) The executive control network stays active to maintain the meditator's focus (vigilance) on the breath. Redrawn from Ricard et al.[38] Copyright © 2020 Kryski Biomedia

these attentional practices also bring additional benefits: regulation of emotional processing, and control and alteration of self-referential processing.

Modulation of Attentional Resources

Mindfulness practices have been demonstrated to enhance the attention system (Figure 5.1), which consists of three functionally distinct but related neural networks.[11] (1) The *alerting network* is involved in achieving and sustaining an alert and aroused state. It is associated with brain activity in the frontoparietal association cortex, the upper brainstem, and diencephalon, as well as levels of norepinephrine in the cortex.[12] (2) The *orienting network* directs and limits attention to a subset of possible inputs. It consists of two subsystems—the dorsal system (frontal eye field and intraparietal sulcus) and the ventral system (temporal-parietal junction in the inferior parietal lobe). The dorsal orienting system is responsible for disengaging and reallocating attention to new perceptual cues.[11,13] When cues are not available, the ventral orienting system is responsible for disengaging attention prior to the presentation of a stimulus.[14] (3) The *executive control network* prioritizes among competing tasks and responses. It consists of two subsystems: the salience network (anterior cingulate cortex and anterior insula) and frontoparietal network (dorsolateral prefrontal cortex). The *salience network* is involved in detecting and monitoring conflicts when a target stimulus must be distinguished and selected from a wide range of competing stimuli,[15] whereas the *frontoparietal network* is responsible for maintaining focus on a selected target.[16]

Mindfulness training has been shown to boost varying aspects of attention, including strengthening selective attention, enhancing vigilance (the ability to sustain attention), decreasing attentional blink, increasing meta-awareness, improving working memory, and improving scores on the Graduate School Entrance (GRE) examination.[17-19] Specifically, open monitoring is associated with enhanced orienting attention and executive control,[18,20] with increased activation of the executive control network—anterior cingulate and dorsolateral prefrontal cortex.[21,22] Furthermore, focused attention improves attentional stability[23] and sustained attention through enhanced executive control,[24] and it produces greater activation of the orienting network in advanced meditators than in novices.[25]

Regulation of Emotional Processing and Control

While a central outcome of attentional practices is changes in the attention networks, converging evidence has shown additional benefits of mindfulness (open monitoring) practice in emotional regulation.[26,27] For example, mindfulness meditation increases biomarkers for well-being and positive affect.[28-30] Additionally, it reduces brain activity in the amygdala—a central node in the limbic system that is associated with emotional reactivity—including reducing amygdala volume[31] and its activation.[22,32,33] Mindfulness practice also increases activation in the prefrontal cortex involved in emotion regulation and the top-down executive inhibition of the amygdala,[34] notably the dorsolateral prefrontal cortex,[35] as well as the dorsomedial prefrontal cortex[33] and the orbitofrontal area in the prefrontal cortex.[36,37] The ability to regulate emotion through mindfulness is a prerequisite for cultivating compassion (feeling *with* the other) in order to counteract the initial negative emotion that one experiences when seeing the suffering of another person (feeling *into* the other).

Alteration of Self-Referential Processing

Mindfulness also modulates *self-referential processing* (i.e., interpreting phenomenon from the "I" perspective to form a narrative) that often leads to negative-charged emotions.[38–40] A key neural network involved in self-referential processing, mind wandering, and ruminative mental activity (e.g., daydreaming, contemplating the future, reliving the past, or general rumination) is the *default mode network*.[41–43] It consists of two major nodes: the medial prefrontal cortex and posterior cingulate cortex.[44] The first node—the medial prefrontal cortex—is subdivided into the ventromedial and dorsomedial prefrontal cortices. The ventromedial prefrontal cortex is interconnected with the amygdala[43–45] and is concerned with emotional processing, whereas the dorsomedial prefrontal cortex is associated with self-referential judgments.[44] The second node—the posterior cingulate cortex (and the medial precuneus)—has dense reciprocal anatomical and functional connections with the hippocampus[43,46] and is associated with recollection of prior experiences,[44] as well as with self-related processes such as "being caught up" in one's experience.[39]

To illustrate the interactions among the default mode network, emotional processing, and memory, let's use a hypothetical scenario in which one is almost hit by a truck when crossing the street (Figure 5.2). In response to this near miss, the amygdala (the "emotor") generates emotions such as fear and anxiety. The hippocampus, being the "memorizer," consolidates this incident into long-term memory. The posterior cingulate cortex (the "selfer"), in turn, adds a sense of self to

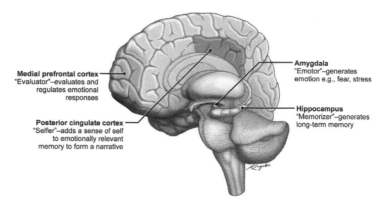

Figure 5.2 Interactions between the default mode network, emotional processing, and memory (see text for details).[38] Copyright © 2020 Kryski Biomedia

emotionally relevant memory to form a narrative (e.g., "I almost get hit by a truck"). The medial prefrontal cortex (the "evaluator") assesses emotional responses and adds meaning to this fearful event. For example, the event could be interpreted as a learning experience which is helpful and adaptive (e.g., "I need to be more careful next time when I cross the street"). Alternatively, because of negativity bias (see Chapter 3), the ordeal could generate a series of unpleasant thoughts (e.g., "I could have been badly injured. I could have died. What will happen to my family if I die?"). These negative thoughts and imagination, in turn, retrigger the amygdala and keep the default mode network active via a vicious cycle, even though one is not in danger anymore. Therefore, a healthy functional balance between the default mode network and other brain systems (e.g., emotion, memory) help us to plan tasks, review past actions, improve future behaviours, and remember pertinent life details. However, if unbalanced, mental unrest including anxiety, obsession, major depression, and other mental illnesses may ensue.[47–50]

Mindfulness practice modulates self-referential processing and mind-wandering through increased functional connectivity between the posterior cingulate cortex and brain regions involved in top-down executive control, working memory, and salience detection (e.g., the anterior cingulate and dorsolateral prefrontal cortex) (Figure 5.3).[51,52] This increase in functional connectivity is associated with reduced stress,[53] negative affect,[54] the experience of pain,[55] and circulating cytokine interluekin-6, a biomarker of inflammation and stress.[51,52] In experienced practitioners, there is also decreased activity in the posterior cingulate cortex which is associated with less self-focus (i.e., more decentring),[56] as well as reduced activity in the medial prefrontal cortex, which is linked to less ruminating activity and less "efforting" required to maintain attentional and emotional stability.[51,57]

In summary, foundational attentional practices in focused attention and open monitoring set the stage for compassion training

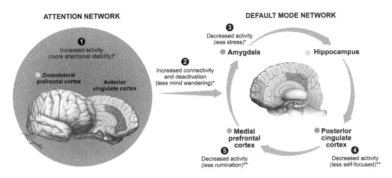

Figure 5.3 Summary of effects of mindfulness meditation on attention, emotional regulation, and self-referential processing. (1) Increased activity in the attention network leads to enhanced attentional stability.[23,24] (2) Increased connectivity between the dorsolateral prefrontal cortex and the default mode network (in particular, the posterior cingulate cortex) leads to deactivation of the default mode network, less mind wandering, and decreased biomarkers of inflammation (e.g., circulating cytokine interluekin-6).[51,52] (3) Down-regulation of activity in the amygdala leads to reduced stress. (4) Decreased activity in the posterior cingulate cortex is associated with less self-focus (i.e., more decentring) in experienced practitioners.[56] (5) Decreased activity in the medial prefrontal cortex in seasoned meditators leads to less ruminating activity and less "efforting" required to maintain attentional and emotional stability[51,57] (* denotes effects seen in both new and seasoned meditators; ** denotes effects seen in seasoned meditators only).[38] Copyright © 2020 Kryski Biomedia

by modulating attentional resources (in the attention networks), regulating emotional processing and control (in the limbic system), and altering self-referential processing (in the default mode network). The ability to modulate self-referential processing is important because self–other discrimination is a crucial mechanism that distinguishes empathic distress from healthy compassion.[58] The changes in self-referential processing through mindfulness practice may, therefore, play a crucial role in compassion and loving-kindness in enhancing one's ability to actively sustain positive other-oriented emotional states and prosocial motivation, which I discuss in the next section.

The Practice of Compassion and Loving-Kindness

Focused attention and open monitoring are foundational skills that strengthen one's ability to maintain focus and develop a sense of equanimity in the face of any positive or negative thoughts, feelings, or sensations that may arise. For this reason, emphasis has been placed mostly on the development of these foundational attentional skills in most Western contemporary mindfulness programs, with the deliberate cultivation of compassion as a central focus being a more recent phenomenon. Indeed, these prerequisite skills are emphasized in both Buddhist[59] and contemporary Western compassion training, such as Compassion Cultivation Training,[60,61] Cognitively Based Compassion Training,[62,63] the ReSource Project,[64] Being with Dying program,[65] and G.R.A.C.E. training.[65–67]

In compassion training, compassion (wishing others to be free from suffering) is typically practised alongside loving-kindness (wishing others to be happy) to further reduce self-concerns and promote positive, other-oriented attitudes. In one common practice (*mettā*), practitioners first bring to mind a loved one, wishing him or her to be happy and free from suffering, and then gradually extend their well-wishes successively to include a friend, a stranger, an enemy, and ultimately all beings, including oneself.[68] In another common practice called "giving and taking" (*tonglen*), practitioners breathe in with the wish to take away the suffering of a specific person and breathe out with the wish to send comfort and happiness to the same person.[69]

The benefits of cultivating compassion have been documented in a number of studies, with two major meta-analyses of randomized clinical trials reported. The first one found that "kindness-based" meditation is moderately effective in increasing compassion, inner compassion, and mindfulness. and in decreasing self-reported depression.[70] In another meta-analysis, compassion-based interventions were again found to have moderate effects on increasing compassion, inner compassion, and mindfulness, and on decreasing depression.[71] In addition, the same meta-analysis reported a reduction in anxiety and psychological distress, as well as an increase in life satisfaction and happiness.[71]

Before I embark on an exploration of the neuroscience of compassion, it is important to note that attentional practices also result in changes in neural circuitry that overlap with those found in loving-kindness/compassion training. For example, similar to attentional practices, loving-kindness/compassion practice also has been shown to suppress activity in the amygdala[51] as well as the default mode network in self-referential processing.[72,73] In addition, while there is a burgeoning body of research on loving-kindness/compassion training, no studies have investigated the neural changes after training in the other immeasurables—sympathetic joy and equanimity. Few emerging studies have examined whether mindfulness practice may increase equanimity or empathic concern and prosocial behaviours; however, it can be argued that these behaviours are quite distinct from the deliberate cultivation of equanimity or loving-kindness/compassion during the cultivation of the four immeasurables. With this in mind, we are now ready to address a central question that I posed earlier: How does the cultivation of loving-kindness and compassion uniquely influence neural processes *above and beyond* those shared with attentional training?

Converging evidence has revealed that loving-kindness and compassion practices lead to three behavioural and neural outcomes: (1) increased receptivity to others' emotions, (2) enhanced positive affect and reward processing, and (3) increased motivation for prosocial connection, including increased motivation to approach others in states of distress.[74-76]

Increased Receptivity to Others' Emotions

Research has shown that compassion/loving-kindness training heightens receptivity and engagement in the emotions of others through modulation of activity in the amygdala of the limbic system. As mentioned in the previous section, the amygdala is a central node in the limbic system in emotional processing and the perception of social information,[77,78] including evaluations of facial expressions for their emotional significance,[79] trustworthiness, and attractiveness.[80] During active compassion meditation, increased activation of both the amygdala[81,82] and its functional connectivity to cortical regions involved in emotion regulation (e.g., the anterior cingulate cortex) has been found.[83] It is interesting to note that this effect is different from the effects of attentional training, which shows *decreased amygdala activity and increased functional connectivity*, as compared to *increased activation of both* during compassion/loving-kindness meditation. This difference could be reconciled by considering that attentional training leads to the *down-regulation of negative affect* (i.e., reduced emotional reactivity), while compassion/loving-kindness practice results in the *up-regulation of positive affect* in response to the emotions of others.[75]

Enhanced Positive Affect and Reward Processing

A recent systematic review and meta-analysis of 24 empirical studies on loving-kindness/compassion practice reported increased positive emotional states in daily life.[84] In addition, brain areas that are involved in pleasure and reward processing (the striatal mesolimbic dopamine system),[85] including romantic love,[86,87] maternal affiliation,[87] and prosocial behaviour,[88] have increased activation during loving-kindness/compassion meditation in both experienced[89] and novice meditators.[58,90-92]

Interestingly, the effects of empathy (feeling *into* others) and com-passion (feeling *with* others) are distinct, both in terms of the af-fect elicited and the neural circuitry involved (Figure 5.4). Empathy training increases negative affect and activates a brain network that is involved in pain processing. In contrast, compassion training increases positive affect (no effect on negative affect) and activates the pleasure and reward system involved in approach and prosocial behaviour.[90] As discussed earlier, empathy can result in two types of responses: empathic distress (i.e., empathic fatigue) and empathic concern. Empathic distress/empathic fatigue refers to a strong aver-sive and self-oriented response to the others' suffering accompanied by the desire to withdraw in order to protect oneself from excessive negative emotion. Empathic concern, on the other hand, is an other-oriented response associated with a sense of warmth, approach, and prosocial motivation that primes compassion. From a neuroscience standpoint, we can now see that the neural mechanisms underlying the two are very different: empathic distress results from *over-stimulation or over-arousal* of the brain network involved in pain processing when witnessing others' suffering, whereas compassion results from acti-vation of the pleasure and reward system while wishing others to be free from suffering. Compassion can thus be viewed as an emotion-regulation strategy that counteracts negative emotion through the ac-tive generation of positive emotion. In this regard, and as discussed in Chapter 1, "compassion fatigue" is a misnomer[93-96] because com-passion does not lead to fatigue; instead, it serves to enhance positive emotion and prosocial behaviour. "Empathy fatigue" is a more ap-propriate term to describe the distress associated with empathy when emotions are not regulated.

Another interesting observation is that *schadenfreude*, or enjoyment of the suffering of others, seems to be quite akin to compassion in that it also activates the pleasure and reward system in response to others' suffering.[98] However, they differ in that *schadenfreude* is accentuated by self-focused states such as envy,[99] whereas compassion/loving-kindness is related to reduced self-concern, which should minimize envy. Future research should measure envy to ensure that the pleasure experienced during compassion/loving-kindness meditation is not caused by self-focused pleasure that results from observing others'

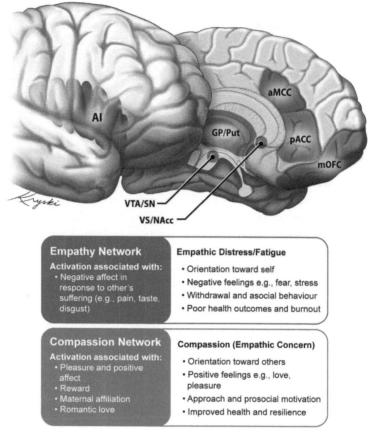

Figure 5.4 Empathy training increases negative affect and activates a brain network that is involved in pain processing (i.e., empathy network—areas shown in pink). In contrast, compassion training increases positive affect (but has no effect on negative affect) and activates the pleasure and reward system that is involved in positive emotion (i.e., compassion network—areas shown in purple). AI, anterior insula; aMCC, anterior mid-cingulate cortex; mOFC, medial orbitofrontal cortex; pACC, pregenual anterior cingulate cortex; GP/Put, globus pallidus/putaman; VS/NAcc, ventral striatum/nucleus accumbens; VTA/SN, ventral tegmental area/substantia nigra. Redrawn from Singer and Klimecki (2014).[97] Copyright © 2020 Kryski Biomedia

suffering, but rather is caused by other-focused pleasure derived from the wish to alleviate others' suffering.[75,98]

Increased Motivation for Prosocial Connection

Compassion/loving-kindness heightens prosocial motivation to connect with others through the modulation of activity in two brain areas: (1) the cognitive executive (e.g., the dorsolateral prefrontal cortex) and emotion control systems and (2) the social bonding and maternal nurturing areas.[91,92,100]

As discussed earlier, negative emotion can overwhelm the capacity to help others[101] and cause empathic distress, whereas compassion practice increases positive affect but has no effect on negative affect.[90] These observations suggest that brain regions involved in the regulation of emotion and cognitive executive control may also play a role in promoting altruistic and prosocial behaviour by increasing the perceived value of helping.[102] Indeed, compassion training increases functional connectivity between regions involved in cognitive executive control (the dorsolateral prefrontal cortex) and reward processing (nucleus accumbens).[103]

Brain areas involved in social bonding and maternal nurturing are also activated after compassion meditation.[91,92,100] Interestingly, these areas are highly sensitive to oxytocin, a hormone known to promote social bonding and maternal nurturing behaviours in human and nonhuman animals.[104] These areas are known to activate the pleasure and reward system, including the periaqueductal gray and septal regions.[87]

In summary, loving-kindness/compassion practices modulate (1) the activity in the *amygdala* involved in detection and appraisal of the emotions of others, (2) the *reward and pleasure system* that may underscore the universal pleasant experience of the immeasurables, (3) the *cognitive executive and emotion control systems* that may help increase the perceived value of helping, and finally, (4) the *social bonding and maternal nurturing areas* involved in parental care of offspring.

Neuroplasticity: Compassion Is Both Innate and a Trainable Skill

Is compassion innate? Can it be learned, taught, and cultivated? The answers to both questions are a resounding yes: compassion is both innate and a trainable skill. As reviewed in this and previous chapters, scientists have mapped out the biological basis of compassion, signifying its deep evolutionary purpose to promote greater proximity, support, and protection among kin (Chapter 1). When we experience compassion, our neuroendocrine system produces oxytocin and vasopressin, while our parasympathetic nervous system, through the ventral vagus nerve, produces a calm, peaceful state. Together, these two physiological systems foster affiliation and bonding (Chapter 2). Psychological research (Chapter 3) also offers us insight into the role that attachment style plays in modulating compassion, as well as the role played by the affiliative system (which facilitates compassion) and the threat and drive systems (which impede it). Taken together, humans have an innate ability for affiliation, compassion, and prosociality.

Consistent with Eastern wisdom traditions, advances in neuroscience demonstrate that not only is compassion innate, it is also a trainable skill (Chapters 4 and 5), exerting its effects through neuroplasticity: the capacity of neurons and neural networks to change their connections—and hence our behaviours—in response to new experience. These neural connections are strengthened further through repeated exposures to the novel experience (i.e., repetitions). Notably, neuroplasticity is not limited only to childhood: the adult brain also possesses a remarkable ability to grow, recover, and adapt. As Dr. Andrew Weil, Clinical Professor of Medicine and Professor of Public Health at the University of Arizona, said: "Neuroplasticity means that emotions such as happiness and compassion can be cultivated in much the same way that a person can learn through repetition to play golf and basketball or master a musical instrument, and that such practice changes the activity and physical aspects of specific brain areas."[105] Reflecting on my own experience, having an understanding of the neural mechanisms underlying compassion training has become a powerful motivator for me to practise meditation. I sometimes even imagine how different parts of my brain are "lighting up" and how new neural connections are being made and reinforced during meditation!

Remarkably, not only is compassion trainable, but the ability to sustain one's attention (i.e., mindfulness)—a foundational practice for the cultivation of compassion—is trainable, too. In our modern world, we are distracted constantly in countless ways. Whether texting, checking emails, answering phone calls, entertainment, or advertisement, these distractions seem to come at us faster, louder, and with an increasing sense of urgency. They beg for our attention and keep us from focusing on what is important. Yet the capacity for sustained voluntary attention is crucial. Great athletes, surgeons, scientists, musicians, mathematicians, and philosophers all exhibit an extraordinary ability to focus their attention for long periods of time. Moreover, mindfulness practice helps decrease self-referential processing and our self-centredness, a state that all major spiritual traditions emphasize. William James (1842–1910), the "Father of American psychology," wrote: "The faculty of voluntarily bringing back a wandering attention over and over again is the very root of judgment, character, and will. . . . An education which would improve this faculty would be the education *par excellence*. But it is easier to define this ideal than to give practical direction for bringing it about."[106] James clearly recognized the importance of the ability to voluntarily sustain one's attention but was not able to provide practical methods for achieving this goal. I imagine that he would be very pleased to learn about the attention training techniques that Eastern contemplative traditions have to offer and the scientific evidence that supports their effectiveness.

Science and the Relative Truth

I would be remiss not to point out that the scientific exposé we have reviewed in the last few chapters is based heavily on the philosophical underpinnings of modern science—namely, scientific realism, reductionism, and materialism[107,108]—that still prevail in many scientific disciplines today despite the discovery of quantum mechanics in the 20th century that have put them into dispute.

The premise of scientific realism is that all matter exists independently in the objective world. Scientific realism assumes that reality is out there waiting to be discovered and is independent of a perceiving agent. However, quantum mechanics has shown that observation alone can affect reality. For instance, all matter exhibits both particle and wave-like properties. In a famous experiment, the very act of introducing an observer altered the behaviour of electrons from that of waves to particles, even though the experimental condition remained identical.[109] In the context of compassion, we may ask: What is the impact of the "act of observing" by the experimenter itself on the neural activity of the meditators when performing neuroimaging experiments? How about gene expression? In addition to environmental and cultural influences, can the expression of the oxytocin gene be controlled by conscious effort?

Further propelling most of Western science, scientific reductionism assumes that all matter and phenomena can be understood by reducing them to smaller basic components. For example, it presupposes that the study of mental functions (e.g., attention, cognition, emotion) can be achieved by conceptually dividing the brain into different systems and subsystems. Similarly, psychology proposes different emotion and behavioural systems to describe the evolution and development of compassion. It is important to remember that while this approach makes complex phenomena easier to understand, it is bound to oversimplify a human experience as rich, sophisticated, and unique as compassion.

Along the same line, scientific materialism assumes that matter is the only fundamental reality. It presupposes that all beings, processes, and phenomena can be explained as manifestations or results of matter. For example, perceptions, thoughts, and emotions are believed to be epiphenomenon of the brain and biological processes. We may ask: Is the activation of the ventral vagal system or the neuroendocrine (oxytocin) system the result of compassion? Or is it the other way round: Is it their activation that leads to the experience of compassion? Or is there a third link; that is, the as yet unknown or poorly understood process called the "mind"?

Although an in-depth comparison of Buddhist philosophy and the philosophy of science is beyond our scope, it is important to note that the Buddhist philosophy of the "Middle Way" takes a very different stance, believing that everything is interdependent, that the way phenomena appear is not the way they exist, and that there are two truths, absolute and relative (phenomenal). In this regard, the science of compassion we explored here could be considered a "relative (phenomenal) truth" that arises from the underlying materialistic, realistic, and reductionistic assumptions that dominate the field of biological science. Nevertheless, from this "relative" perspective, it is fascinating to see the consistency between the 2,500 years of Buddhist practice of loving-kindness and compassion on the one hand and the relevant brain networks and their plasticity in response to training on the other.

One final thought. As with any scientific investigations, the neuroscientific evidence presented here suggests a correlation, rather than causation. We need to be cautious not to equate correlations between brain activities and mental functions with the mind itself. As William James pointed out: "Evidence for mind–brain correlations may indeed imply that the brain produces mental events, or that it has the lesser role of simply releasing or permitting them, or that it merely transmits them, as light hits a prism, thereby transmitting a spectrum of colors."[108] Is compassion simply an epiphenomenon of brain activities, or is it an aspect of the mind? We can go even further: What is awareness and the subjective experience of awareness? Is there a "self"? What is consciousness? What is the mind? Where do they come from? Is the mind an "emergent, self-organizing, embodied, and relational process that regulates the flow of energy and information," as proposed by the noted contemporary American thinker Dr. Daniel Siegel?[110] These are all intriguing questions that certainly give us plenty of food for thought.

Summary of Key Points

- Many contemporary secular compassion training programs are based on the Buddhist teachings that mindfulness is the attentional foundation of compassion practice.
- Mindfulness is based on two foundational contemplative skills: focused attention and open monitoring. Focused attention

directs the mind to focus firmly and exclusively on a single point (e.g., the breath), whereas open monitoring anchors the mind to the present while broadening it to encompass the whole flux of internal and external experiences as they arise and pass away from moment to moment.

- Focused attention and open monitoring set the stage for compassion training by modulating attentional resources (in the attention networks), regulating emotion processing and control (in the limbic system), and altering self-referential processing (in the default mode network).

- The attention system consists of three networks: (1) the alerting network, which sustains an aroused state; (2) the orienting network, which (re)directs and limits attention to a subset of possible inputs; and (3) the executive control network, which consists of two subsystems—the salience network (anterior cingulate cortex and anterior insula), which selects the relevant target, and the frontoparietal network (dorsolateral prefrontal cortex), which maintains focus on the selected target.

- A key neural network involved in self-referential processing, mind-wandering, and ruminative mental activity is the default mode network. A well-balanced default mode network helps us to plan tasks, review past actions, improve future behaviours, and remember pertinent life details. However, if left unchecked, it causes mental unrest, such as anxiety, obsession, major depression, and other mental illnesses.

- Loving-kindness and compassion practices lead to benefits that are above and beyond those that result from mindfulness training. These practices increase one's receptivity to others' emotions (in the limbic system), enhance positive affect and reward processing (in the mesolimbic dopamine system), and increase motivation for prosocial connection (in the cognitive executive and emotion control systems, as well as in the social bonding and maternal nurturing areas).

- "Compassion fatigue" is a misnomer because the neural mechanisms underlying empathic distress and compassion are distinct. Empathic distress results from *over-stimulation or over-arousal* of the brain network involved in pain processing when witnessing others' suffering, whereas compassion results from activation of the pleasure and reward system while wishing others to be free from suffering. "Empathy fatigue" is a more appropriate term to describe the distress associated with empathy when emotions are not regulated. Compassion does not lead to fatigue; instead, it serves as an emotion-regulation strategy that counteracts negative emotion through the active generation of positive emotion to enhance prosocial behaviour.

- Compassion is both innate and trainable, exerting its effect through neuroplasticity. Similar to other skills, both compassion and the capacity to sustain one's attention can be learned and strengthened through repetition to alter the activities in specific brain areas.

References

1. Ñāṇamoli Bhikkhu, Bodhi Bhikkhu. *The Middle Length Discourses of the Buddha: A Translation of the Majjhima Nikaya.* Somerville, MA: Wisdom Publications; 1995.
2. Anālayo Bhikkhu. *Satipaṭṭhāna: The Direct Path to Realization.* Cambridge: Windhorse Publications; 2003.
3. Shankman R. *The Experience of Samadhi: An In-depth Exploration of Buddhist.* Boston, MA: Shambhala Publications; 2008.
4. Ñānananda Bhikkhu. *Concept and Reality in Early Buddhist Thought: An Essay on "Papañca" and "Papañca-Saññā-Saṇkhā."* Kandy, Sri Lanka: Buddhist Publication Society; 1971.
5. Lutz A, Dunne JD, Davidson RJ. Meditation and the neuroscience of consciousness: An Introduction. In: Zelazo P, Moscovitch M, Thompson E, eds. *The Cambridge Handbook of Consciousness.* Cambridge: Cambridge University Press; 2006:499–554.
6. Dunn BR, Hartigan JA, Mikulas WL. Concentration and mindfulness meditations: Unique forms of consciousness? *Appl Psychophysiol Biofeedback.* 1999;24(3):147–165.
7. Brown KW, Ryan RM. The benefits of being present: Mindfulness and its role in psychological well-being. *J Pers Soc Psychol.* 2003;84(4):822–848.
8. Van Vugt MK. Cognitive benefits of mindfulness meditation. In: Brown KW, Creswell JD, Ryan RM, eds. *Handbook of Mindfulness: Theory, Research, and Practice.* New York: Guilford; 2015:190–207.

9. Brown KW, Goodman RJ, Ryan RM, Analayo B. Mindfulness enhances episodic memory performance: Evidence from a multimethod investigation. *PLoS One.* 2016;11(4):e0153309.

10. Atkinson RC, Shiffrin RM. Human memory: A proposed system and its controlprocesses. *Psychol Learn Motiv.* 1968;2:89–195.

11. Petersen SE, Posner MI. The attention system of the human brain: 20 years after. *Annu Rev Neurosci.* 2012;35:73–89.

12. Blumenfeld H. *Neuroanatomy Through Clinical Cases.* Cary, NC: Oxford University Press; 2018.

13. Posner MI, Petersen SE. The attention system of the human brain. *Annu Rev Neurosci.* 1990;13:25–42.

14. Fan J, McCandliss BD, Sommer T, Raz A, Posner MI. Testing the efficiency and independence of attentional networks. *J Cogn Neurosci.* 2002;14(3):340–347.

15. Menon V, Uddin LQ. Saliency, switching, attention and control: A network model of insula function. *Brain Struct Funct.* 2010;214(5–6):655–667.

16. Carter CS, van Veen V. Anterior cingulate cortex and conflict detection: An update of theory and data. *Cogn Affect Behav Neurosci.* 2007;7(4):367–379.

17. Mrazek MD, Franklin MS, Phillips DT, Baird B, Schooler JW. Mindfulness training improves working memory capacity and GRE performance while reducing mind wandering. *Psychol Sci.* 2013;24(5):776–781.

18. Jha AP, Krompinger J, Baime MJ. Mindfulness training modifies subsystems of attention. *Cogn Affect Behav Neurosci.* 2007;7(2):109–119.

19. Goleman D, Davidson RJ. *Altered Traits: Science Reveals How Meditation Changes Your Mind, Brain, and Body.* New York: Penguin Random House; 2017.

20. Tang YY, Ma Y, Wang J, et al. Short-term meditation training improves attention and self-regulation. *Proc Natl Acad Sci U S A.* 2007; 104(43):17152–17156.

21. Baerentsen KB, Hartvig NV, Stødkilde-Jørgensen H, Mammen J. Onset of meditation explored with fMRI. *NeuroImage.* 2001;13(6 Suppl):297.

22. Farb NA, Segal ZV, Mayberg H, et al. Attending to the present: Mindfulness meditation reveals distinct neural modes of self-reference. *Soc Cogn Affect Neurosci.* 2007;2(4):313–322.

23. Lutz A, Slagter HA, Rawlings NB, Francis AD, Greischar LL, Davidson RJ. Mental training enhances attentional stability: Neural and behavioral evidence. *J Neurosci.* 2009;29(42):13418–13427.

24. MacLean KA, Ferrer E, Aichele SR, et al. Intensive meditation training improves perceptual discrimination and sustained attention. *Psychol Sci.* 2010;21(6):829–839.

25. Brefczynski-Lewis JA, Lutz A, Schaefer HS, Levinson DB, Davidson RJ. Neural correlates of attentional expertise in long-term meditation practitioners. *Proc Natl Acad Sci U S A.* 2007;104(27):11483–11488.

26. Tang YY, Holzel BK, Posner MI. The neuroscience of mindfulness meditation. *Nat Rev Neurosci.* 2015;16(4):213–225.
27. Desbordes G, Gard T, Hoge EA, et al. Moving beyond mindfulness: Defining equanimity as an outcome measure in meditation and contemplative research. *Mindfulness.* 2014;6(2):356–372.
28. Urry HL, Nitschke JB, Dolski I, et al. Making a life worth living: Neural correlates of well-being. *Psychol Sci.* 2004;15(6):367–372.
29. Moyer CA, Donnelly MP, Anderson JC, et al. Frontal electroencephalographic asymmetry associated with positive emotion is produced by very brief meditation training. *Psychol Sci.* 2011; 22(10):1277–1279.
30. Barnhofer T, Chittka T, Nightingale H, Visser C, Crane C. State effects of two forms of meditation on prefrontal EEG asymmetry in previously depressed individuals. *Mindfulness.* 2010;1(1):21–27.
31. Taren AA, Creswell JD, Gianaros PJ. Dispositional mindfulness co-varies with smaller amygdala and caudate volumes in community adults. *PLoS One.* 2013;8(5):e64574.
32. Goldin PR, Gross JJ. Effects of mindfulness-based stress reduction (MBSR) on emotion regulation in social anxiety disorder. *Emotion.* 2010;10(1):83–91.
33. Farb NA, Anderson AK, Mayberg H, Bean J, McKeon D, Segal ZV. Minding one's emotions: Mindfulness training alters the neural expression of sadness. *Emotion.* 2010;10(1):25–33.
34. Quirk GJ, Beer JS. Prefrontal involvement in the regulation of emotion: Convergence of rat and human studies. *Curr Opin Neurobiol.* 2006;16(6):723–727.
35. Creswell JD, Way BM, Eisenberger NI, Lieberman MD. Neural correlates of dispositional mindfulness during affect labeling. *Psychosom Med.* 2007;69(6):560–565.
36. Way BM, Creswell JD, Eisenberger NI, Lieberman MD. Dispositional mindfulness and depressive symptomatology: Correlations with limbic and self-referential neural activity during rest. *Emotion.* 2010;10(1):12–24.
37. Zeidan F, Emerson NM, Farris SR, et al. Mindfulness meditation-based pain relief employs different neural mechanisms than placebo and sham mindfulness meditation-induced analgesia. *J Neurosci.* 2015;35(46):15307–15325.
38. Ricard M, Lutz A, Davidson RJ. Mind of the meditator. *Sci Am.* 2014;311(5):38–45.
39. Brewer JA, Garrison KA, Whitfield-Gabrieli S. What about the "self" is processed in the posterior cingulate cortex? *Front Hum Neurosci.* 2013;7:647.
40. Northoff G, Heinzel A, de Greck M, Bermpohl F, Dobrowolny H, Panksepp J. Self-referential processing in our brain: A meta-analysis of imaging studies on the self. *Neuroimage.* 2006;31(1):440–457.

41. Raichle ME, MacLeod AM, Snyder AZ, Powers WJ, Gusnard DA, Shulman GL. A default mode of brain function. *Proc Natl Acad Sci U S A.* 2001;98(2):676–682.

42. Mason MF, Norton MI, Van Horn JD, Wegner DM, Grafton ST, Macrae CN. Wandering minds: The default network and stimulus-independent thought. *Science.* 2007;315(5810):393–395.

43. Vago DR, Silbersweig DA. Self-awareness, self-regulation, and self-transcendence (S-ART): A framework for understanding the neurobiological mechanisms of mindfulness. *Front Hum Neurosci.* 2012;6:296.

44. Raichle ME. The brain's default mode network. *Annu Rev Neurosci.* 2015;38:433–447.

45. Ongur D, Price JL. The organization of networks within the orbital and medial prefrontal cortex of rats, monkeys and humans. *Cereb Cortex.* 2000;10(3):206–219.

46. Vincent JL, Snyder AZ, Fox MD, et al. Coherent spontaneous activity identifies a hippocampal-parietal memory network. *J Neurophysiol.* 2006;96(6):3517–3531.

47. Zidda F, Andoh J, Pohlack S, et al. Default mode network connectivity of fear- and anxiety-related cue and context conditioning. *Neuroimage.* 2018;165:190–199.

48. Bessette KL, Jenkins LM, Skerrett KA, et al. Reliability, convergent validity and time invariance of default mode network deviations in early adult major depressive disorder. *Front Psychiatry.* 2018;9:244.

49. Koch K, Reess TJ, Rus OG, et al. Increased default mode network connectivity in obsessive-compulsive disorder during reward processing. *Front Psychiatry.* 2018;9:254.

50. Reuveni I, Bonne O, Giesser R, et al. Anatomical and functional connectivity in the default mode network of post-traumatic stress disorder patients after civilian and military-related trauma. *Hum Brain Mapp.* 2016;37(2):589–599.

51. Brewer JA, Worhunsky PD, Gray JR, Tang YY, Weber J, Kober H. Meditation experience is associated with differences in default mode network activity and connectivity. *Proc Natl Acad Sci U S A.* 2011;108(50): 20254–20259.

52. Creswell JD, Taren AA, Lindsay EK, et al. Alterations in resting-state functional connectivity link mindfulness meditation with reduced interleukin-6: A randomized controlled trial. *Biol Psychiatry.* 2016;80(1):53–61.

53. Cisler JM, James GA, Tripathi S, et al. Differential functional connectivity within an emotion regulation neural network among individuals resilient and susceptible to the depressogenic effects of early life stress. *Psychol Med.* 2013;43(3):507–518.

54. Goldin PR, McRae K, Ramel W, Gross JJ. The neural bases of emotion regulation: Reappraisal and suppression of negative emotion. *Biol Psychiatry.* 2008;63(6):577–586.

55. Wager TD, Rilling JK, Smith EE, et al. Placebo-induced changes in FMRI in the anticipation and experience of pain. *Science*. 2004;303(5661):1162–1167.

56. Garrison KA, Santoyo JF, Davis JH, Thornhill TAt, Kerr CE, Brewer JA. Effortless awareness: Using real time neurofeedback to investigate correlates of posterior cingulate cortex activity in meditators' self-report. *Front Hum Neurosci*. 2013;7:440.

57. Taylor VA, Grant J, Daneault V, et al. Impact of mindfulness on the neural responses to emotional pictures in experienced and beginner meditators. *Neuroimage*. 2011;57(4):1524–1533.

58. Klimecki OM, Leiberg S, Lamm C, Singer T. Functional neural plasticity and associated changes in positive affect after compassion training. *Cereb Cortex*. 2013;23(7):1552–1561.

59. Sayadaw U Pandita. *In This Very Life*. Boston, MA: Wisdom Publications; 1992.

60. Jazaieri H, Jinpa TL, McGonigal K, Rosenberg E, Finkelstein J, Simon-Thomas E. Enhancing compassion: A randomized controlled trial of a compassion cultivation training program. *J Happiness Stud*. 2013;14:1113–1126.

61. Jazaieri H, Lee I, McGonigal K, et al. A randomized controlled trial of compassion cultivation training: Effects on mindfulness, affect, and emotion regulation. *Motiv Emot*. 2013;38:23–35.

62. Ozawa-de Silva B, Dodson-Lavelle B. An education of heart and mind: Practical and theoretical issues in teaching cognitively based compassion training to children. *Practical Matters*. 2011;4:1–28.

63. Negi LT. *Emory Compassion Meditation Protocol: Cognitively-Based Compassion Training Manual*. Atlanta, GA: Emory University; 2013.

64. Singer T, Kok BE, Bornemann B, Zurborg S, Bolz M, Bochow C. *The ReSource Project: Background, Design, Samples, and Measurements* (2nd ed.). Leipzig: Max Planck Institute for Human Cognitive and Brain Sciences; 2016.

65. Rushton CH, Sellers DE, Heller KS, Spring B, Dossey BM, Halifax J. Impact of a contemplative end-of-life training program: Being with dying. *Palliat Support Care*. 2009;7(4):405–414.

66. Halifax J. G.R.A.C.E. for nurses: Cultivating compassion in nurse/patient interactions. *J Nurse Educ Pract*. 2014;4(1):121–128.

67. Halifax J. A heuristic model of enactive compassion. *Curr Opin Support Palliat Care*. 2012;6(2):228–235.

68. Salzberg S. *Real Love: The Art of Mindful Connection*. New York: Flatiron Books; 2017.

69. Chödrön P. *How to Meditate: A Practical Guide to Making Friends with Your Mind*. Boulder, CO: Sounds True; 2013.

70. Galante J, Galante I, Bekkers MJ, Gallacher J. Effect of kindness-based meditation on health and well-being: A systematic review and meta-analysis. *J Consult Clin Psychol*. 2014;82(6):1101–1114.

71. Cultivating compassion: A systematic review and meta-analysis of compassion-based interventions. PROSPERO: International Prospective Register of Systematic Reviews, 2015, CRD42015024576. 2015. http://www.crd.york.ac.uk/PROSPERO/display_record.asp?ID= CRD42015024576

72. Garrison KA, Scheinost D, Constable RT, Brewer JA. BOLD signal and functional connectivity associated with loving kindness meditation. *Brain Behav.* 2014;4(3):337–347.

73. Garrison KA, Zeffiro TA, Scheinost D, Constable RT, Brewer JA. Meditation leads to reduced default mode network activity beyond an active task. *Cogn Affect Behav Neurosci.* 2015;15(3):712–720.

74. Stevens L, Benjamin J. The brain that longs to care for others: The current neuroscience of compassion. In: Stevens L, Woodruff CC, eds. *The Neuroscience of Empathy, Compassion, and Self-Compassion.* London: Academic Press, Elsevier; 2018:53–89.

75. Goodman RJ, Plonski PE, Savery L. Compassion training from an early Buddhist perspective: The neurological concomitants of the brahmavihāras. In: Stevens L, Woodruff CC, eds. *The Neuroscience of Empathy, Compassion, and Self-Compassion.* London: Academic Press, Elsevier; 2018: 235–266.

76. Flasbeck V, Gonzalez-Liencres C, Brune M. The brain that feels into others: Toward a neuroscience of empathy. In: Stevens L, Woodruff CC, eds. *The Neuroscience of Empathy, Compassion, and Self-Compassion.* London: Academic Press, Elsevier; 2018:23–51.

77. Mosher CP, Zimmerman PE, Gothard KM. Neurons in the monkey amygdala detect eye contact during naturalistic social interactions. *Curr Biol.* 2014;24(20):2459–2464.

78. Pessoa L, Adolphs R. Emotion processing and the amygdala: From a "low road" to "many roads" of evaluating biological significance. *Nat Rev Neurosci.* 2010;11(11):773–783.

79. Sato W, Yoshikawa S, Kochiyama T, Matsumura M. The amygdala processes the emotional significance of facial expressions: An fMRI investigation using the interaction between expression and face direction. *Neuroimage.* 2004;22(2):1006–1013.

80. Bzdok D, Langner R, Hoffstaedter F, Turetsky BI, Zilles K, Eickhoff SB. The modular neuroarchitecture of social judgments on faces. *Cereb Cortex.* 2012;22(4):951–961.

81. Lutz A, Brefczynski-Lewis J, Johnstone T, Davidson RJ. Regulation of the neural circuitry of emotion by compassion meditation: Effects of meditative expertise. *PLoS One.* 2008;3(3):e1897.

82. Desbordes G, Negi LT, Pace TW, Wallace BA, Raison CL, Schwartz EL. Effects of mindful-attention and compassion meditation training on amygdala response to emotional stimuli in an ordinary, non-meditative state. *Front Hum Neurosci.* 2012;6:292.

83. Leung MK, Chan CC, Yin J, Lee CF, So KF, Lee TM. Enhanced amygdala-cortical functional connectivity in meditators. *Neurosci Lett.* 2015;590:106–110.

84. Zeng X, Chiu CP, Wang R, Oei TP, Leung FY. The effect of loving-kindness meditation on positive emotions: A meta-analytic review. *Front Psychol.* 2015;6:1693.

85. Phan KL, Wager T, Taylor SF, Liberzon I. Functional neuroanatomy of emotion: A meta-analysis of emotion activation studies in PET and fMRI. *Neuroimage.* 2002;16(2):331–348.

86. Aron A, Fisher H, Mashek DJ, Strong G, Li H, Brown LL. Reward, motivation, and emotion systems associated with early-stage intense romantic love. *J Neurophysiol.* 2005;94(1):327–337.

87. Bartels A, Zeki S. The neural correlates of maternal and romantic love. *Neuroimage.* 2004;21(3):1155–1166.

88. Harbaugh WT, Mayr U, Burghart DR. Neural responses to taxation and voluntary giving reveal motives for charitable donations. *Science.* 2007;316(5831):1622–1625.

89. Engen HG, Singer T. Compassion-based emotion regulation up-regulates experienced positive affect and associated neural networks. *Soc Cogn Affect Neurosci.* 2015;10(9):1291–1301.

90. Klimecki OM, Leiberg S, Ricard M, Singer T. Differential pattern of functional brain plasticity after compassion and empathy training. *Soc Cogn Affect Neurosci.* 2014;9(6):873–879.

91. Kim JW, Kim SE, Kim JJ, et al. Compassionate attitude towards others' suffering activates the mesolimbic neural system. *Neuropsychologia.* 2009;47(10):2073–2081.

92. Beauregard M, Courtemanche J, Paquette V, St-Pierre EL. The neural basis of unconditional love. *Psychiatry Res.* 2009;172(2):93–98.

93. Hofmeyer A, Kennedy K, Taylor R. Contesting the term "compassion fatigue": Integrating findings from social neuroscience and self-care research. *Collegian.* 2019;27(2):232–237.

94. Dowling T. Compassion does not fatigue! *Can. Vet. J.* 2018;59(7): 749–750.

95. Ricard M. *Altruism: The Power of Compassion to Change Yourself and the World.* New York: Little, Brown and Company; 2015.

96. Halifax J. *Standing at the Edge.* New York: Martin's Press; 2018.

97. Singer T, Klimecki OM. Empathy and compassion. *Curr Biol.* 2014;24(18):R875–R878.

98. West TN, Savery L, Goodman RJ. Sometimes I get so mad I could. . . . The neuroscience of cruelty. In: Stevens L, Woodruff CC, eds. *The Neuroscience of Empathy, Compassion, and Self-Compassion.* London: Academic Press, Elsevier; 2018:121–155.

99. Takahashi H, Kato M, Matsuura M, Mobbs D, Suhara T, Okubo Y. When your gain is my pain and your pain is my gain: Neural correlates of envy and schadenfreude. *Science.* 2009;323(5916):937–939.

100. Morelli SA, Rameson LT, Lieberman MD. The neural components of empathy: Predicting daily prosocial behavior. *Soc Cogn Affect Neurosci.* 2014;9(1):39–47.

101. Cameron CD, Payne BK. Escaping affect: How motivated emotion regulation creates insensitivity to mass suffering. *J Pers Soc Psychol.* 2011;100(1):1–15.

102. Ochsner KN, Gross JJ. The cognitive control of emotion. *Trends Cogn Sci.* 2005;9(5):242–249.

103. Weng HY, Fox AS, Shackman AJ, et al. Compassion training alters altruism and neural responses to suffering. *Psychol Sci.* 2013;24(7):1171–1180.

104. Rilling JK. The neural and hormonal bases of human parental care. *Neuropsychologia.* 2013;51(4):731–747.

105. Weil A. *Spontaneous Healing: How to Discover and Enhance Your Body's Natural Ability to Maintain and Heal Itself.* New York: Knopf; 1995.

106. James W. *The Principles of Psychology.* New York: Dover Publications; 1950.

107. Wallace BA. *The Taboo of Subjectivity: Toward a New Science of Consciousness.* New York: Oxford University Press; 2004.

108. Wallace BA. *Buddhism with an Attitude: The Tibetan Seven-Point Mind Training.* Ithaca, NY: Snow Lion Publications; 2003.

109. Buks E, Schuster R, Heiblum M, Mahalu D, Umansky V. Dephasing in electron interference by a "which-path" detector. *Nature.* 1998;391:871–874.

110. Siegel DJ. *Mind: A Journey to the Heart of Being Human.* New York: W. W. Norton & Company; 2016.

6

What Are the Obstacles
to Compassion?

Compassion is a complex process that is influenced by a number of conscious and unconscious factors. Indeed, there are many examples in which psychological factors, beliefs, values, context, organizational culture, and societal forces have led to harm from lack of compassion (acts of omission) and hostility (acts of commission). In this chapter, I examine some of the obstacles that impede the flow of compassion in three directions: for others, from others, and from self (Figure 6.1). I also discuss the barriers to compassion that are unique in the health-care environment.

Obstacles to Compassion for Others

As discussed in Chapter 3, attachment style affects compassion, especially in those with insecure attachment during early development. Avoidant individuals are uncomfortable with distress and may distance themselves from other's suffering. They may also view support seekers as weak and become contemptuous toward others in distress.[1] Anxiously attached individuals, in contrast, can become overly helpful in order to be liked.[1]

Another factor is personal identity. For example, high masculine identity, especially when linked to a loss of poise in helping, suppresses prosocial behaviours.[2] Similarly, individuals with a low moral self-identity exhibit less favourable attitudes toward aiding out-group members.[3]

Compassion can be inhibited when it is being perceived as detrimental to self-interests.[4] People who are motivated by high social dominance—that is, those who view the world as a competitive,

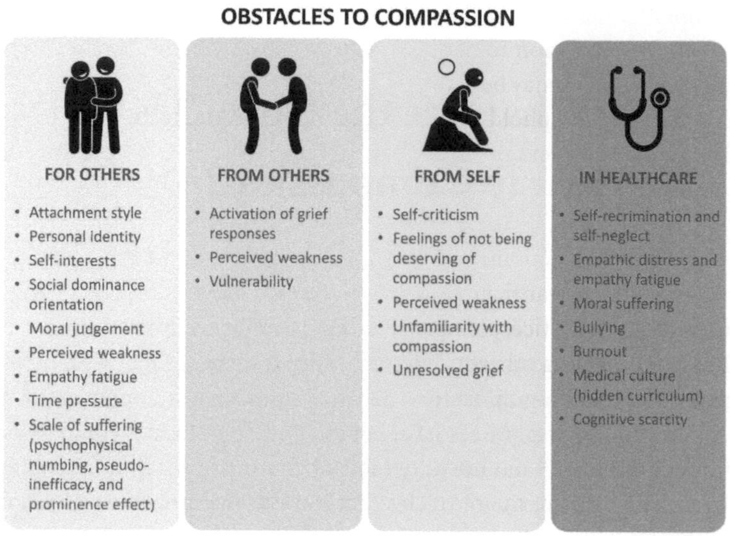

OBSTACLES TO COMPASSION

FOR OTHERS	FROM OTHERS	FROM SELF	IN HEALTHCARE
• Attachment style • Personal identity • Self-interests • Social dominance orientation • Moral judgement • Perceived weakness • Empathy fatigue • Time pressure • Scale of suffering (psychophysical numbing, pseudo-inefficacy, and prominence effect)	• Activation of grief responses • Perceived weakness • Vulnerability	• Self-criticism • Feelings of not being deserving of compassion • Perceived weakness • Unfamiliarity with compassion • Unresolved grief	• Self-recrimination and self-neglect • Empathic distress and empathy fatigue • Moral suffering • Bullying • Burnout • Medical culture (hidden curriculum) • Cognitive scarcity

Figure 6.1 Obstacles to compassion for others, from others, from self, and in healthcare.

dog-eat-dog environment of winners and losers—can endorse very noncompassionate values to out-groups.[5,6] They are more ruthless, less other-concerned, less tolerant, and often linked to the dark triad of Machiavellianism (manipulation, deception, and exploitation), narcissism, and psychopathy.[6–8] Driven by an up-rank mentality, those with high social dominance orientation strive for leadership positions, and, when they become leaders, they are willing to use unethical means such as exploitation to achieve economic, social, and political gains.[9,10] Alarmingly, the negative effect of social dominance orientation on empathy over time is stronger than the positive effect of empathy on social dominance orientation over time.[5] This may help explain the corrosive effect of this style of leadership on institutional norms and personal integrity. Indeed, motivated by the desire to protect one's self-interest, severe lapses in compassion have been seen repeatedly in history in normally kind and upright people who try to fit in, carry out orders, or follow group disciplines for self-preservation.[11]

Moral judgment may also play a role. When people perceive the receiver of compassion to have committed a moral injustice, empathy-induced altruism may be inhibited. Indeed, empathy-induced altruism and the wish to uphold a moral principle, such as a principle of justice, are independent prosocial motives that sometimes cooperate but sometimes conflict.[12]

Confusing compassion as a sign of submissiveness or weakness may hinder prosocial actions. In studies of retributive versus restorative justice, people can fear that compassion can be perceived as prioritizing sympathy over justice, condoning bad behaviours, letting offenders off the hook, enabling others to take advantage of one's kindness and forgiveness, or being irrational.[13]

Compassion can also be reduced to a self-focused emotional state. For example, traumatized individuals, including those who are overworked or vicariously traumatized, can experience empathy fatigue that can lead to selfish prosocial or self-focused behaviours rather than the healthy empathic concern that primes compassion.[14] In addition, efforts to be compassionate could be hazardous to health when caring is viewed as mandatory and when the perceived needs exceed available resources.[15]

Time pressure is another barrier to compassion. For instance, in the famous "Good Samaritan Study," seminary students were told that they needed to prepare a brief sermon about the Good Samaritan from the Bible. They were instructed to walk to a nearby building to give their sermon and were either told that they were early, on-time, or running late. While on their way, all participants encountered an injured stranger, who was an actor planted by the researchers, in a narrow alleyway. The researchers found that time-constraint mattered—63% in the "early" group and 45% in the "on-time" group stopped to help the stranger, in contrast to only 10% in the "late" group.[16] These results powerfully demonstrate how busyness, hurrying, and distraction can affect our ability to notice or engage in compassionate action.

The scale of suffering also has an enormous impact on people's willingness to help. Three psychological obstacles that inhibit response to major crises have been identified. *Psychophysical numbing* refers to the observation that, as the number of victims in a tragedy increases, the more apathy ensues.[17] It may result from diminished sensitivity to

the value of life or our inability to appreciate losses of life as they become larger.[17] Another obstacle is *pseudo-inefficacy*, a demotivation to
help because of an illusion of ineffectiveness.[18] For example, the money
donated to a 7-year-old African child facing starvation decreased
dramatically when the donor was made aware that the child was one
of millions needing food aid.[19] The third obstacle is the *prominence
effect*: people prefer options that are easy to justify and defend.[20] For
example, at the government level, we often see the prominence effect
of economic or security interests supersede the decision to intervene,
stop, or prevent a mass atrocity. Indeed, the recent covid-19 pandemic
illustrates vividly how these three obstacles—psychophysical numbing,
pseudo-inefficacy, and the prominence effect of economic interests—
affect our responses as we witnessed the appallingly high toll of deaths
and suffering not only locally but also around the world.

Obstacles to Receiving Compassion
from Others and Self

Receiving compassion from others and especially from self can be
difficult in modern contemporary culture.[21] For some individuals,
the feelings of kindness associated with compassion from others
can activate grief responses—of wanting but not obtaining the care
and warmth one needs from early supportive attachment figures,
with a heightened experience of loneliness and a longing for close
relationships.[22] They may also view receiving compassion as a sign of
weakness and not be willing to be in a vulnerable position when they
are in distress.

For some people, inner compassion—the ability to turn understanding, acceptance, and love inward toward self—is often met with
doubt, fear, and resistance.[21] It is linked to feelings of not being deserving of compassion, a weakness, unfamiliarity with compassion,
and unresolved grief of wanting love and kindness but often feeling
lonely and rejected.[23] This resistance can be prominent, especially in
individuals who come from a background where there is abuse or little
affection.[24] A lack of inner compassion has been linked to difficulties
with receiving compassion from others, and both are associated with

self-criticism, self-coldness, insecure attachment, stress, anxiety, and depression.[25]

A major obstacle to inner compassion is self-criticism (self-judgment, self-contempt, self-disparagement, and self-attack),[26,27] which is found in many who work in healthcare (a topic that I explore further in the next section on self-recrimination and self-neglect). *Self-criticism* is the evaluation of one's own behaviours and attributes, with recognition of one's weaknesses, errors, and shortcomings.[28] It is characterized by negative evaluations of the self, often involving internal self-talk that is highly negative, disparaging, and berating.[29] It often involves unhelpful thinking styles that use first-person (I am . . .) or second-person (you are . . .) statements and include labelling (making global and pejorative statements about oneself based on a behaviour in a particular situation, such as "I am an idiot"); inflexibility/unyielding (using "should" statements to put unreasonable expectations or pressure on oneself, such as "you should have known better"); and overgeneralizing (drawing a broad, general conclusion from one negative instance that is not supported by available evidence, such as "it will never work").[29]

The typical threat that often lurks behind self-criticism, as well as behind many difficult, unresolved, and recurring emotions, is a sense of shame—"being seen as, or experiencing oneself as, incompetent, useless, ugly, undesired, unwanted" and fear of "social criticism or even attack, disconnection, being marginalized, unloved, and unwanted; and at times weak and defenceless."[22,27] In fact, according to psychologist Paul Gilbert, self-criticism and shame are the two most prevalent problems in mental health.[27,30]

Factors that contribute to self-criticism are varied. Individuals with insecure attachment may be more prone to self-criticism. Self-criticism may also occur in those who lack awareness of their self-critical thinking style or are not recognizing consciously that they are struggling. Positive beliefs about self-criticism as a way of self-improvement may also play a role. Some people use self-criticism as an attempt at self-improvement/self-correction (e.g., a means to address flaws, stop mistakes, better or motivate oneself) or as way of punishment (e.g., to atone for what they have done or their perceived self-image as being bad).[29] Still others may have negative beliefs about inner compassion and use self-criticism as a defense. They fear they would become self-pitying, self-centred, complacent, or under-achieved,[27] all of which are not supported by empirical research.[31]

The self-critical (vicious) cycle is illustrated in Figure 6.2. Triggers, such as a particular situation that one is in, thoughts about the future, and memory of a negative event in the past, as well as uncomfortable feelings or bodily sensations, can quickly and automatically shift the mind into the threat mode. When the threat system is activated,

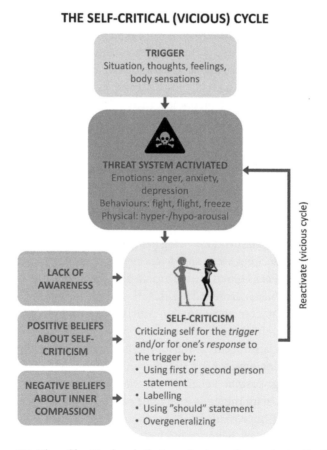

Figure 6.2 The self-critical cycle that reactivates and perpetuates the threat system. Redrawn from Saulsman et al.[29]

a number of unpleasant emotional (anger, anxiety, depression), behavioural (fight, flight, or freeze), and physical (hyper-/hypoarousal) responses follow. Many people deal with perceived threats via self-criticism, either criticizing oneself for the original trigger or one's response to the trigger. Self-criticism is, in turn, supported by a lack of awareness of one's self-critical thinking style, positive beliefs about self-criticism, and negative beliefs about inner compassion. However, self-criticism only serves to reactivate and perpetuate the threat system so that the unpleasant emotional, behavioural, and physical responses persist.[29] The affiliative system is suppressed, and compassion is inhibited.[22]

Obstacles to Compassion in Healthcare

Caring for the health and well-being of others is an intrinsically compassionate behaviour. Compassion is a core value among healthcare workers who have often undergone extensive training to dedicate a major part of their lives to caring for others. However, there are many barriers to compassion despite their best intention.

Self-Recrimination and Self-Neglect

Many healthcare professionals are drawn to the caring professions at least in part because of their own wounds (the "wounded healer" archetype). Their wounds may come from childhood neglect and abuse, parental divorce, significant losses, physical or emotional traumas, poverty, hunger, physical injury and diseases, mental illnesses, addictions, difficult events or situations, betrayals of trust, immigration, or discrimination—in essence, the human condition. The wounded caregivers who are self-aware can better identify, understand, and empathize with the suffering of their patients—relationships that can be mutually transformative. They recognize that their motivation to care for others arises partly from a need to feel loved and existentially secured. However, if they are not aware of their old wounds and past experiences and "sacrifice" themselves in the name of patient care, they can pay a steep price by neglecting their own needs. They may not eat appropriately, work out, take up a hobby, or spend time for self-reflection, regarding these activities as selfish behaviours. They may handle their anxiety or dejection by working even more, drinking, smoking, or using drugs.[32] This self-neglect and isolation, together with self-recrimination, self-doubt, and guilt and exacerbated by a medical culture that demands stoicism and rationality, make for an unhealthy mix that, over time, can lead to a dearth of compassion toward self that in turn affects caring for others.

Empathic Distress and Empathy Fatigue

Healthcare workers are expected to be empathetic and compassionate in caring for patients. Empathy improves clinical outcomes,[33] patient satisfaction and compliance,[34] as well as professional satisfaction.[35] Although empathy is trainable, it is often considered a "fluffy" skill in medical education, with very little emphasis being placed on its cultivation. It is disheartening to see that numerous studies have shown that empathy decreases during medical/nursing school and residency while cynicism increases.[36-38] Without empathy/compassion training, it is perhaps not surprising that caregivers find it challenging to regulate their responses to human suffering, with negative consequences for both patients and their families.

When healthcare workers encounter a distressing event, such as witnessing the suffering of another or endeavouring to alleviate another's suffering, the emotions they experience depend on their individual attributes. These attributes include the ability to attune to others emotionally (empathy), cognitively (perspective-taking), and ethically (moral sensitivity). They can also become attuned through memory, such as personal and professional experiences, cultural or societal experiences, personal and familial history, core values, and professional culture (Figure 6.3).[14,39] If these attributes are aligned, empathic arousal may evoke a positive emotional response through positive emotion regulation, resulting in healthy empathic concern that leads to compassionate action. When these attributes are not aligned, however, empathic arousal may result in negative emotions, such as

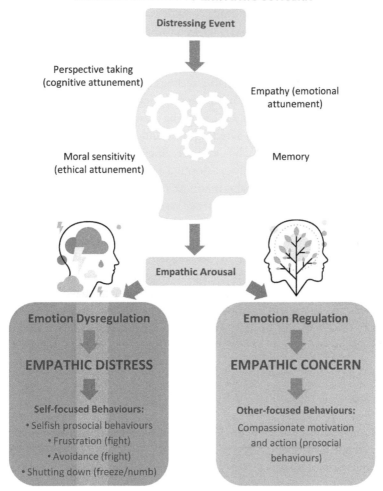

Figure 6.3 A model of empathic arousal through emotion regulation that leads to empathic distress versus empathic concern. Modified from Baston et al.,[40] Eisenberg et al.,[39,50] and Rushton et al.[14]

sorrow, guilt, regret, frustration, or anger. When negative empathic arousal becomes overwhelming, emotional dysregulation may result, leading to empathic distress, an aversive emotional reaction.[39–41] To cope with empathic distress, individuals may engage in self-focused behaviours, such as selfish prosocial behaviours that aim primarily to relieve one's own uncomfortable feelings rather than the suffering of another (e.g., rushing to comfort another who is crying). Self-focused behaviours also include fight (e.g., being frustrated or adopting a combative style), flight (e.g., avoiding or abandoning patients physically, emotionally, or spiritually), and freezing/numbing responses (e.g., shutting down emotionally or adopting a stoic demeanor).

Personal distress may also manifest itself as unregulated actions, including burnout and moral outrage (see next sections). Additionally, healthcare professionals may suffer in response to repeated exposure or re-exposure to the suffering and trauma of others resulting in vicarious trauma.[42] They may also experience symptoms similar to posttraumatic stress disorder without having necessarily been exposed to direct trauma themselves (i.e., secondary traumatic stress).[43] Indeed, empathy fatigue and secondary traumatic stress have been recognized as a "cost of caring" and a key contributor to the loss of compassion in healthcare.[43,44]

Moral Suffering

Central to healthcare is the ability to make difficult decisions in the face of ethical dilemmas, yet healthcare professionals receive very little education in bioethics. Without training, individuals may lack *moral sensitivity*, the ability to recognize morally pertinent features and identify moral conflicts, as well as *moral discernment*, the ability to evaluate which actions are morally admissible.[45] When confronted with morally distressing situations, they may become confused, agitated, or frustrated because they lack the vocabulary and training to articulate and process their experience.

Moral suffering is the distress experienced in response to moral harms, wrongs, or failures. It includes moral distress, moral injury, moral outrage, and moral apathy.[45] *Moral distress* is the experience of knowing the right thing to do but not being able to do so because of internal or external constraints,[46] such as when a healthcare team is being compelled to initiate or continue futile life support at a family's insistence, or when patients are discharged because of lack of beds despite knowing that they will not receive adequate support in the community. Moral distress has been correlated with empathic distress, secondary traumatic stress, and burnout.[47,48] Healthcare workers may experience *moral remainder*, a painful emotional residue that lingers after being forced to choose between two or more deeply held beliefs or values.[49]

Moral injury, on the other hand, is a complex psychological, social, cultural, and spiritual injury to an individual's moral conscience resulting from witnessing or participating in an act of perceived moral transgression.[51] It is often associated with shame, guilt, withdrawal, depression, self-loathing, and alienation. Alarmingly high incidences of moral injury have been reported in a number of nursing areas including critical care, emergency, oncology, pediatric, mental health, and midwifery.[43] For example, intensive care nurses experience moral injury or secondary traumatic stress triggered by situations that may include seeing patients die, large open wounds, massive bleeding, trauma-related injuries, care futility, patient aggression, and involvement with end-of-life care, as well as being subjected to verbal abuse from family members, physicians, and other nurses.[52] Physicians may experience moral injury when they provide suboptimal care because of pressures from administrators or insurers to reduce cost. Healthcare leaders may experience moral injury when, despite disagreement, they have to carry out administrative decisions or policies that they consider short-sighted, harmful, or in conflict with their personal values.

Healthcare givers may also experience *moral outrage*—a constellation of cognitive, affective, and behavioural responses—that arises from anger and disgust when one recognizes that a person or institution has violated a moral principle.[53] For example, they may become enraged when they witness poor patient care as a result of a lack of provider continuity or team communication. Healthcare leaders may encounter moral outrage when they deal with peers, hospital administrators, or system bureaucrats who are unprofessional, duplicitous, or incompetent. Principled moral outrage can be beneficial by motivating one to take the right action and bring about changes. However, when it is unexamined or driven by unmet (often unconscious) needs, indignation, or self-righteousness, moral outrage can become contagious, escalate conflicts, and perpetuate the drama triangle of persecutor, victim, and rescuer.[54]

Opposite to moral outrage, caregivers may experience *moral apathy* when they become indifferent, willfully disregard, or deny or seal themselves off from the suffering of others or harmful situations,[45] such as when they keep quiet while witnessing others' behaviours that are unsafe, incompetent, or harmful.

From a larger perspective, what is rarely discussed is the importance that healthcare professionals develop a strong moral character, the ability to attain and maintain moral integrity and to act in alignment with their ethical values. It involves having the strength and courage to sustain one's convictions, persisting and overcoming distractions and obstacles, and implementing skills to do the right thing. It arises from training of the mind, emotions, and behaviours that uphold important ethical values. The prevailing bioethics model, however, focuses on adherence to principles—autonomy, justice, beneficence, and nonmaleficence. An important question is: How do we cultivate ethics as a practice to explore and discover our own biases, with the intention of bringing about compassion, relationality, moral sensitivity, integrity, patience, trust, humility, and an ability to accept ambivalence?

Bullying

For many healthcare workers, a lack of respect and compassion in the form of bullying is a common experience.[55,56] Bullying entails both *horizontal hostility,* which occurs between people of equal rank, and *vertical violence,* which happens between people of different rank. It includes rude, ignoring, humiliating behaviours; yelling; snide comments; and withholding pertinent information. In a recent survey of 7,887 doctors in the United Kingdom, 40% reported that bullying, harassment, or undermining is an issue in their workplace.[57] Bullying is also widespread in nursing, with a prevalence upward of 80%.[55,56] A recent review of 79 papers in the nursing literature revealed that bullying is a predictor of burnout, that bullied nurses recorded 1.5 times higher absenteeism compared to the non-bullied group, and that 78.5% of bullied nurses with length of service less than 5 years resigned from their job.[55]

The causes of bullying are many and complex. Many, especially those in training or more junior positions, are often reluctant to report incidents of bullying. Many who have been bullied or harassed are often targeted because they are isolated or in a weak position. They fear repercussions and find it difficult to challenge this behaviour because it often comes from the top. To make matters worse, their colleagues do not speak up either, allowing such behaviour to go unchallenged, become normalized, and form part of the culture. This collective silence is further exacerbated by the lack of clarity on what is acceptable behaviour, the lack of commitment or training of departmental heads and managers to handle the problem, and the lack of an effective complaints and resolution process.

Unfortunately, ignoring bullying comes at a heavy cost to both individuals and organizations, as well as to patient care and safety (e.g., by withholding needed information or creating an adversarial environment). Those who have been bullied say they struggled to function and felt physically sick and emotionally broken. It affected their families, destroyed their confidence, and caused lasting harm to their careers.[57] Up to 75% of the victims reported psychological disturbances ranging from irritability and insomnia, to psychosomatic symptoms, posttraumatic stress disorders, and, in some cases, suicide ideation.[58-60]

Burnout

Many healthcare professionals are engaged, energized, and feel nourished by their work. They have a sense of personal agency and believe that their work makes a difference. Engagement, however, can slip into *burnout*: a depleted state characterized by emotional exhaustion, depersonalization, and low personal accomplishment.[61,62] What contributes to burnout? While many have asserted erroneously that burnout and professional satisfaction are solely the responsibility of the individual, many studies have pointed out that the local work environment is a major stressor.[63-65] In primary care practices, poor workflow (time pressure and a chaotic and inefficient work environment in which physicians are required inappropriately to perform clerical and other mundane tasks), low work control (over work conditions and decision-making), and unfavourable organizational culture have been found to be associated strongly with low physician satisfaction, high stress, and burnout.[64] For surgical practices, a survey of 7,905 surgeons found that factors that are associated independently with burnout include younger age, having children, subspecialty choice, high number of nights on call per week, high number of hours worked per week, and having compensation based entirely on billing or productivity.[65] Importantly, these studies found that physician satisfaction is linked primarily to their relationship with patients rather than compensation[64] and that physicians who spend more than 20% of their time on what they consider the most meaningful activity are least prone to burnout.[66] High prevalence of burnout has also been reported among nurses: emotional exhaustion was found in 31%, depersonalisation in 24%, and low personal accomplishment in 38% of nurses.[67] Factors related to burnout in nursing include professional experience (junior nurses) and marital status (being single), as well as psychological and workplace factors (multiple employments, work overload).[67]

Other stressors that contribute to burnout and that act as barriers to compassion in healthcare include the fear of making errors,[68,69] time pressure,[70,71] role confusion or conflicts,[72-74] poor levels of staffing,[75] job insecurity,[67] complex clinical situations,[76] poor leadership,[77] and excessive/defensive bureaucracy.[78]

Medical Culture

Last, I would like to discuss two phenomena that are unique to physicians: medical culture and cognitive scarcity. Medicine has its own culture with distinct standards of behaviours, evaluation, and values, as well as beliefs, myths, and symbols.[79] The medical socialization process begins as one enters medical school, a rite of passage during which one has little control over one's life.[80] Medical students are under enormous pressure to memorize voluminous amounts of information and master technical skills. When they become residents and fellows, they work long hours, have more responsibility, and fear making mistakes, all exacerbated by sleep deprivation and social isolation. They worry about being humiliated when failing to answer a question at grand rounds, thus feeling ashamed of their imperfect knowledge. They are busy surviving, dealing with multiple competing priorities. They have limited mental resources to reflect on and sustain their personal values and sense of purpose. Yet these inner resources are not only crucial as they witness human suffering, fear, ambiguity, uncertainty, and death, but also necessary to support their own well-being.

Physicians-in-training also have little time to challenge the legitimacy of what they are learning or ponder about the system of power and hierarchy that they are experiencing. While the "official curriculum" formally stipulates the set of knowledge and skills required of physicians, the medical culture also strongly influences the values and behaviours of future doctors through unofficial and implicit modes of socialization—the so-called *hidden curriculum*.[81] It consists of unexamined practices (e.g., a doctor should not show emotions, especially negative ones), assumptions (e.g., training requires sacrifice), rules (e.g., trainees should just do the work and not complain), protocols (e.g., don't challenge your superiors), power, privileges, domination (e.g., using pejorative humor toward certain types of patients that one may have deemed offensive before medical school), and indifference to discrimination (detachment from or cynicism toward patients).[79] In the face of this hidden curriculum, many trainees feel silenced or powerless when confronted with power hierarchy, unethical, or even harmful behaviours. The hidden curriculum is also a main reason for empathy decline during medical school and residency.[36,38]

With the advent of evidence-based medicine, the practice and teaching of medicine further reinforce a reductionist scientific paradigm at the expense of the cultivation of the values, principles, and practice of caregiving. Evidence-based medicine de-emphasizes intuition and unsystematic clinical experience as valuable tools for clinical decision-making, favouring instead the use of biomedical evidence from clinical research.[82] Although in recent years the definition of evidence-based medicine has been revised and improved as an approach to integrate clinical expertise and patient values with the best available research evidence,[83] a reductionistic and detached approach continues to prevail. For example, during many formal and informal trainings/discussions, patients are often reduced to as "cases" or statistics, without much attention given to address the personhood of the afflicted or their condition and struggle, especially when clinicians are under time pressure.

Although both Canada and the United States recently adopted competency-based models,[84] formal training remains largely dedicated to two traditional competencies—medical expert and scholar—with very little curricular time assigned to the five so-called "soft skills": communication, collaboration, leadership, advocacy, and professionalism.[85] Added to the problem is that many physician-educators are not familiar with how to teach or assess these skills. The biggest challenge is that, with the current medical philosophy that is predominantly quantitative, empirical, and reductionist, how do we teach and measure qualities such as deep listening, informed intuition, intersubjectivity, human caring, benevolence, and cultural sensitivity, with all their complexity, richness, and depth?

Cognitive Scarcity

In addition to clinical decisions, physicians nowadays also need to evaluate the financial consequences of their decisions on patients and their fiscal responsibility to the healthcare system as its gatekeepers to ration or deny healthcare. *Cognitive scarcity* refers to the dissonance and dilemma that physicians experience when they have to make decisions that have difficult tradeoffs and consequential outcomes (i.e., opportunity costs). Evidence has shown that when people have to deliberate on the opportunity costs of each of their decisions, their cognitive performance on logic and problem-solving tasks declines significantly.[86] The current intense focus on economic rationality, with its imperative to contain cost, maximize productivity, and enhance efficiency,[87] is not what physicians are trained in nor is it what draws them to medicine in the first place. Economic rationality deprives physicians of the moral experience of doctoring—to restore health and alleviate human suffering—that sustains, energizes, and engages them.[88] It is perhaps not surprising that physician burnout, suboptimal care, and lack of compassion, as well as a decline in humanity and moral values are some of the unintended outcomes of modern healthcare. How can we return healthcare back to its original fundamental core—a deeply interpersonal, relational practice that resonates with physicians, other healthcare professionals, and patients through compassionate care?[89] What concrete steps can we take to cultivate compassion not only in our individual lives, but also in the ailing healthcare system? We will discuss these questions in the next chapter.

Summary of Key Points

- Obstacles to compassion for others include insecure attachment style, personal identity, self-interests, social dominance orientation, moral judgment, confusing compassion with submissiveness or weakness, empathy fatigue, time pressure, and scale of suffering (including psychophysical numbing, pseudo-inefficacy, and prominence effect).
- Obstacles to receiving compassion from others include activation of grief responses, perceived weakness, and vulnerability.
- Obstacles to receiving compassion from self (inner compassion) include feelings of not being deserving of compassion, weakness, unfamiliarity with compassion, unresolved grief, and self-criticism.
- Self-criticism is characterized by negative evaluations of the self and internal self-talk that is highly negative, disparaging, and berating. It involves unhelpful thinking styles that include labelling, inflexibility/unyielding, and overgeneralizing.
- Factors that contribute to self-criticism include insecure attachment style, lack awareness of self-critical thinking style, positive beliefs about self-criticism as a way of self-improvement or self-punishment, using self-criticism as a defense, and negative beliefs about inner compassion (i.e., confusing inner compassion with self-pitying, self-centredness, complacency, or under-achieving).

- Obstacles to compassion in healthcare include self-recrimination and self-neglect ("wounded healer"), empathic distress and empathy fatigue, moral suffering, bullying, burnout, medical culture (hidden curriculum), and cognitive scarcity.
- Empathic distress is an aversive reaction that occurs when emotional arousal is not regulated. It leads to self-focused actions which include selfish prosocial behaviours, fight, flight, and freezing/numbing responses.
- Moral suffering includes moral distress, moral injury, moral outrage, and moral apathy. *Moral distress* is the experience of knowing the right thing to do but not being able to do so because of internal or external constraints. *Moral injury* occurs when one witnesses or participates in an act of perceived moral transgression that results in injury to one's moral conscience. *Moral outrage* is the anger and disgust that arise when one recognizes that a person or institution has violated a moral principle. *Moral apathy* occurs when one becomes indifferent to the suffering of others that results from the violation of a moral principle.
- Bullying entails both horizontal hostility, which occurs between people of equal rank, and vertical violence, which happens between people of different rank. It includes rude, ignoring, and humiliating behaviours; yelling; snide comments; and withholding pertinent information.
- Burnout is a depleted state characterized by emotional exhaustion, depersonalization, and low personal accomplishment. It is not solely the responsibility of the individual because local work environment and systemic issues are major contributing factors.

References

1. Mikulincer M, Shaver PR, Gillath O, Nitzberg RA. Attachment, caregiving, and altruism: Boosting attachment security increases compassion and helping. *J Pers Soc Psychol.* 2005;89(5):817–839.
2. Tice DM, Baumeister RF. Masculinity inhibits helping in emergencies: Personality does predict the bystander effect. *J Pers Soc Psychol.* 1985;49:420–428.

3. Reed A, 2nd, Aquino KF. Moral identity and the expanding circle of moral regard toward out-groups. *J Pers Soc Psychol.* 2003;84(6):1270–1286.
4. Gerhardt S. *The Selfish Society: How We All Forgot to Love One Another and Made Money Instead.* London: Simon & Schuster; 2010.
5. Sidanius J, Kteily N, Sheehy-Skeffington J, Ho AK, Sibley C, Duriez B. You're inferior and not worth our concern: The interface between empathy and social dominance orientation. *J Pers.* 2013;81(3):313–323.
6. Pratto F, Sidanius J, Stallworth LM, Malle BF. Social dominance orientation: A personality variable predicting social and political attitudes. *J Pers Soc Psychol.* 1994;67:741–763.
7. Furnham A, Richards SC, Paulhus DL. The dark triad of personality: A 10 year review. *Soc Personal Psychol Compass.* 2013;7:199–221.
8. Duckitt J. A dual-process cognitive-motivational theory of ideology and prejudice. *Adv Exp Soc Psychol.* 2001;33:41–113.
9. Altemeyer B. What happens when authoritarians inherit the earth? A simulation. *Anal Soc Issues Public Policy.* 2003;3(1):161–169.
10. Son Hing LS, Bobocel DR, Zanna MP, McBride MV. Authoritarian dynamics and unethical decision making: High social dominance orientation leaders and high right-wing authoritarianism followers. *J Pers Soc Psychol.* 2007;92(1):67–81.
11. Kelman HC, Hamilton VL. *Crimes of Obedience.* New Haven, CT: Yale University Press; 1989.
12. Batson CD, Klein TR, Highberger L, Shaw LL. Immorality from empathy-induced altruism: When compassion and justice conflict. *J Pers Soc Psychol.* 1995;68:1042–1054.
13. McLaughlin E, Huges G, Fergusson R, Westmarland L. *Restorative Justice: Critical Issues.* London: Sage; 2003.
14. Rushton CH, Kaszniak AW, Halifax JS. A framework for understanding moral distress among palliative care clinicians. *J Palliat Med.* 2013;16(9):1074–1079.
15. Vitaliano PP, Zhang J, Scanlan JM. Is caregiving hazardous to one's physical health? A meta-analysis. *Psychol Bull.* 2003;129(6):946–972.
16. Darley JM, Batson CD. From Jerusalem to Jericho: A study of Situational and Dispositional Variables in Helping Behavior. *J Pers Soc Psychol.* 1973;27:100–108.
17. Fetherstonhaugh D, Slovic P, Johnson SM, Friedrich J. Insensitivity to the value of human life: A study of psychophysical numbing. *J Risk Uncertain.* 1997;14(3):283–300.
18. Västfjäll D, Slovic P, Mayorga M. Whoever saves one saves the world: Confronting the challenge of pseudo-inefficacy. 2014. https://cpb-us-e1.wpmucdn.com/blogs.uoregon.edu/dist/6/6757/files/2014/07/Whoever-Saves-One-Life-Saves-the-World-1wda5u6.pdf

19. Small DA, Loewenstein G, Slovic P. Sympathy and callousness: The impact of deliberative thought on donations to identifiable and statistical victims. *Organ Behav Hum Decis Process.* 2007;102:143–153.

20. Slovic P. Choice between equally valued alternatives. *J Exp Psychol Hum Percept Perform.* 1975;1:280–287.

21. Jinpa T. *A Fearless Heart: How the Courage to Be Compassionate Can Transform Our Lives.* New York: Hudson Street Press; 2015.

22. Gilbert P. The origins and nature of compassion focused therapy. *Br J Clin Psychol.* 2014;53(1):6–41.

23. Gilbert P, Procter S. Compassionate mind training for people with high shame and self-criticism: Overview and pilot study. *Clin Psychol Psychother.* 2006;13:353–379.

24. Mikulincer M, Shaver PR. *Attachment in Adulthood: Structure, Dynamics, And Change.* New York: Guilford; 2007.

25. Gilbert P, McEwan K, Matos M, Rivis A. Fears of compassion: Development of three self-report measures. *Psychol Psychother.* 2011;84(3):239–255.

26. Dunkley DM, Zuroff DC, Blankstein KR. Self-critical perfectionism and daily affect: Dispositional and situational influences on stress and coping. *J Pers Soc Psychol.* 2003;84(1):234–252.

27. Gilbert P, Irons C. Focused therapies and compassionate mind training for shame and self-attacking. In: Gilbert P, ed. *Compassion: Conceptualisations, Research and Use in Psychotherapy.* New York: Routledge; 2005:263–325.

28. APA Dictionary of Psychology. 2018. https://dictionary.apa.org/self-criticism

29. Saulsman L, Campbell B, Sng A. Building self-compassion: From self-criticism to self-kindness. Perth, Western Australia Centre for Clinical Interventions; 2017: https://www.cci.health.wa.gov.au/Resources/Looking-After-Yourself/Self-Compassion

30. Low CA, Schauenburg H, Dinger U. Self-criticism and psychotherapy outcome: A systematic review and meta-analysis. *Clin Psychol Rev.* 2020;75:101808.

31. Barnard LK, Curry JF. Self-compassion: Conceptualizations, correlates, & interventions. *Rev Gen Psychol* 2011;15(4):289–303.

32. Myers MF. *Why Physicians Die by Suicide.* New York: Michael F Myers; 2017.

33. Di Blasi Z, Harkness E, Ernst E, Georgiou A, Kleijnen J. Influence of context effects on health outcomes: A systematic review. *Lancet.* 2001;357(9258):757–762.

34. Kim SS, Kaplowitz S, Johnston MV. The effects of physician empathy on patient satisfaction and compliance. *Eval Health Prof.* 2004;27(3):237–251.

35. Bertakis KD, Roter D, Putnam SM. The relationship of physician medical interview style to patient satisfaction. *J Fam Pract.* 1991;32(2):175–181.

36. Neumann M, Edelhauser F, Tauschel D, et al. Empathy decline and its reasons: A systematic review of studies with medical students and residents. *Acad Med.* 2011;86(8):996–1009.
37. Ward J, Cody J, Schaal M, Hojat M. The empathy enigma: An empirical study of decline in empathy among undergraduate nursing students. *J Prof Nurs.* 2012;28(1):34–40.
38. Hojat M, Vergare MJ, Maxwell K, et al. The devil is in the third year: A longitudinal study of erosion of empathy in medical school. *Acad Med.* 2009;84(9):1182–1191.
39. Eisenberg N, Fabes RA, Murphy B, et al. The relations of emotionality and regulation to dispositional and situational empathy-related responding. *J Pers Soc Psychol.* 1994;66(4):776–797.
40. Batson CD, Fultz J, Schoenrade PA. Distress and empathy: Two qualitatively distinct vicarious emotions with different motivational consequences. *J Pers.* 1987;55(1):19–39.
41. Eisenberg N. Distinctions among various modes of empathy-related reactions: A matter of importance in humans. *Behav Brain Sci.* 2002;25:33–34.
42. Pearlman LA, Saakvitne KW. Treating therapists with vicarious traumatization and secondary traumatic stress disorders. In: Figley CR, ed. *Compassion Fatigue: Coping with Secondary Traumatic Stress Disorder in Those Who Treat the Traumatized.* New York: Brunner/Mazel; 1995:150–177.
43. Missouridou E. Secondary posttraumatic stress and nurses' emotional responses to patient's trauma. *J Trauma Nurs.* 2017;24(2):110–115.
44. Sinclair S, Raffin-Bouchal S, Venturato L, Mijovic-Kondejewski J, Smith-MacDonald L. Compassion fatigue: A meta-narrative review of the healthcare literature. *Int J Nurs Stud.* 2017;69:9–24.
45. Halifax J. *Standing at the Edge.* New York: Martin's Press; 2018.
46. Jameton A. *Nursing Practice: The Ethical Issues.* Englewood Cliffs, NJ: Prentice-Hall; 1984.
47. Austin CL, Saylor R, Finley PJ. Moral distress in physicians and nurses: Impact on professional quality of life and turnover. *Psychol Trauma.* 2017;9(4):399–406.
48. Oh Y, Gastmans C. Moral distress experienced by nurses: A quantitative literature review. *Nurs Ethics.* 2015;22(1):15–31.
49. Tessman L. *When Doing the Right Thing Is Impossible.* New York: Oxford University Press; 2017.
50. Eisenberg N. Empathy-related emotional responses, altruism, and their socialization. In: Davidson R, Harrington A, eds. *Visions of Compassion: Western Scientists and Tibetan Buddhists Examine Human Nature.* New York: Oxford University Press; 2002:131–164.

51. Litz BT, Stein N, Delaney E, et al. Moral injury and moral repair in war veterans: A preliminary model and intervention strategy. *Clin Psychol Rev.* 2009;29(8):695–706.

52. Mealer ML, Shelton A, Berg B, Rothbaum B, Moss M. Increased prevalence of post-traumatic stress disorder symptoms in critical care nurses. *Am J Respir Crit Care Med.* 2007;175(7):693–697.

53. Salerno JM, Peter-Hagene LC. The interactive effect of anger and disgust on moral outrage and judgments. *Psychol Sci.* 2013;24(10):2069–2078.

54. Karpman SB. *A Game Free Life. The Definitive Book on the Drama Triangle and Compassion Triangle by the Originator and Author. The New Transactional Analysis of Intimacy, Openness, and Happiness.* San Francisco: Drama Triangle Publications; 2014.

55. Bambi S, Foa C, De Felippis C, Lucchini A, Guazzini A, Rasero L. Workplace incivility, lateral violence and bullying among nurses. A review about their prevalence and related factors. *Acta Biomed.* 2018;89(6-S):51–79.

56. Wilson JL. An exploration of bullying behaviours in nursing: A review of the literature. *Br J Nurs.* 2016;25(6):303–306.

57. British Medical Association. Future vision for the NHS: All member survey. https://www.bma.org.uk/collective-voice/policy-and-research/nhs-structure-and-delivery/future-vision-forthe-nhs/future-vision-for-the-nhs-survey Published 2018.

58. Dumont C, Meisinger S, Whitacre MJ, Corbin G. Nursing 2012. Horizontal violence survey report. *Nursing.* 2012;42(1):44–49.

59. Edwards SL, O'Connell CF. Exploring bullying: Implications for nurse educators. *Nurse Educ Pract.* 2007;7(1):26–35.

60. Bambi S, Guazzini A, De Felippis C, Lucchini A, Rasero L. Preventing workplace incivility, lateral violence and bullying between nurses: A narrative literature review. *Acta Biomed.* 2017;88(5S):39–47.

61. Maslach C, Jackson SE. The measurement of experienced burnout. *J Organ Behav.* 1981;2:99–113.

62. Freudenberger HJ. Staff Burn-out. *J Soc Issues.* 1974;30:159–165.

63. Shanafelt TD, Noseworthy JH. Executive leadership and physician well-being: Nine organizational strategies to promote engagement and reduce burnout. *Mayo Clin Proc.* 2017;92(1):129–146.

64. Linzer M, Manwell LB, Williams ES, et al. Working conditions in primary care: Physician reactions and care quality. *Ann Intern Med.* 2009;151(1):28–36, W26–29.

65. Shanafelt TD, Balch CM, Bechamps GJ, et al. Burnout and career satisfaction among American surgeons. *Ann Surg.* 2009;250(3):463–471.

66. Shanafelt TD, West CP, Sloan JA, et al. Career fit and burnout among academic faculty. *Arch Intern Med.* 2009;169(10):990–995.

67. Molina-Praena J, Ramirez-Baena L, Gomez-Urquiza JL, Canadas GR, De la Fuente EI, Canadas-De la Fuente GA. Levels of burnout and risk factors

in medical area nurses: A meta-analytic study. *Int J Environ Res Public Health.* 2018;15(12).

68. Robertson JJ, Long B. Suffering in silence: Medical error and its impact on health care providers. *J Emerg Med.* 2018;54(4):402–409.

69. Vrbnjak D, Denieffe S, O'Gorman C, Pajnkihar M. Barriers to reporting medication errors and near misses among nurses: A systematic review. *Int J Nurs Stud.* 2016;63:162–178.

70. Vinckx MA, Bossuyt I, Dierckx de Casterle B. Understanding the complexity of working under time pressure in oncology nursing: A grounded theory study. *Int J Nurs Stud.* 2018;87:60–68.

71. Rabatin J, Williams E, Baier Manwell L, Schwartz MD, Brown RL, Linzer M. Predictors and outcomes of burnout in primary care physicians. *J Prim Care Community Health.* 2016;7(1):41–43.

72. Gray FC, White A, Brooks-Buck J. Exploring role confusion in nurse case management. *Prof Case Manag.* 2013;18(2):66–76; quiz 77–68.

73. Tarrant T, Sabo CE. Role conflict, role ambiguity, and job satisfaction in nurse executives. *Nurs Adm Q.* 2010;34(1):72–82.

74. Tunc T, Kutanis RO. Role conflict, role ambiguity, and burnout in nurses and physicians at a university hospital in Turkey. *Nurs Health Sci.* 2009;11(4):410–416.

75. Mannion R. Enabling compassionate healthcare: Perils, prospects and perspectives. *Int J Health Policy Manag.* 2014;2(3):115–117.

76. de Zulueta PC. Developing compassionate leadership in health care: An integrative review. *J Healthc Leadersh.* 2016;8:1–10.

77. West MA, Chowla R. Compassionate leadership for compassionate health care. In: Gilbert P, ed. *Compassion. Concepts, Research and Applications.* New York: Routledge; 2017:237–257.

78. Cole-King A, Gilbert P. Compassionate care: The theory and the reality. *J Holistic Healthcare.* 2011;8(3):29–37.

79. Vaidyanathan B. Professional socialization in medicine. *AMA J Ethics.* 2015;17(2):164–170.

80. Peterkin AD. *Staying Human During Residency Training: How to Survive and Thrive After Medical School* (6th ed.). Toronto: University of Toronto Press; 2016.

81. Hafferty FW. Beyond curriculum reform: Confronting medicine's hidden curriculum. *Acad Med.* 1998;73(4):403–407.

82. Evidence-Based Medicine Working Group. Evidence-based medicine. A new approach to teaching the practice of medicine. *JAMA.* 1992;268(17):2420–2425.

83. Masic I, Miokovic M, Muhamedagic B. Evidence based medicine: New approaches and challenges. *Acta Inform Med.* 2008;16(4):219–225.

84. Frank JR, Snell L, Sherbino J, eds. *CanMEDS 2015 Physician Competency Framework.* Ottawa: Royal College of Physicians and Surgeons of Canada; 2015.

85. Peterkin AD, Skorzewska A, eds. *Health Humanities in Postgraduate Medical Education.* New York: Oxford University Press; 2018.
86. Mani A, Mullainathan S, Shafir E, Zhao J. Poverty impedes cognitive function. *Science.* 2013;341(6149):976–980.
87. Berwick DM, Nolan TW, Whittington J. The triple aim: Care, health, and cost. *Health Aff (Millwood).* 2008;27(3):759–769.
88. Kleinman   A.   Caregiving   as   moral   experience.   *Lancet.* 2012;380(9853):1550–1551.
89. Wong AM. Beyond burnout: Looking deeply into physician distress. *Can J Ophthalmol.* 2020;55(suppl):7–16. doi:10.1016/j.jcjo.2020.01.014.

7

What Does It Take to Cultivate Compassion?

Positive Disintegration and the Edge States

The many challenges and obstacles to compassion that we encounter can be viewed as "positive disintegration"[1]: the stress, anxiety, and crises that we face are important opportunities for our personal growth, maturation, and transformation. Roshi Joan Halifax coined the term "edge states" to describe the internal and interpersonal virtuous qualities and their associated shadow sides that can cause us to "fall off the cliff."[2] When we find ourselves on the precipice—on the high side of edge states such as empathic concern, integrity, and wholesome engagement—we can stand firm there and enjoy the panoramic view, recognizing our contribution to humanity while at the same time having the humility to know that we can lose balance easily and fall off the edge.[2] And if we do fall, we can use the fall as a place of transformation where great potential resides. We can work our way back to the high edge skilfully and nonjudgmentally, cultivating a wider and more inclusive perspective, developing stronger resilience, and opening the gift of compassion to others and ourselves.

What are some of the skills that could help us to cultivate compassion in our daily life? At the personal level, taking care of one's basic needs such as having enough sleep, a balanced diet, regular exercise, and cultivating nourishing relationships that contribute to one's sense of stability, authenticity, and wholeness are crucial. Taking a pause, even for one breath, is also a simple and readily available resource for us to stay grounded despite the busyness of our lives. It allows our mind and body to relax, creates space to refocus our attention, and enables us to perceive more clearly what is happening at this moment so that we can truly serve. As Victor Frankl, an Austrian neurologist, psychiatrist, and Holocaust survivor, said: "Between stimulus and response, there is a space. In that space is our power to choose our response. In our response lies our growth and our freedom."[3]

Training in the development of cognitive, attentional, affective, and somatic skills is also critical. In this regard, contemplative traditions offer many time-tested and skilful approaches for the development and maintenance of compassion, a sense of resilience, and equanimity.[4,5] These skills include awareness practices that help one recognize somatic responses and emotional arousal; mindfulness practices that stabilize attention, monitor thoughts, and regulate emotions; insight practices that develop one's capacity to pause, listen, inquire, explore, and reflect with openness and curiosity; compassion training that primes kindness, generosity, patience, gratitude, and other prosocial attributes; and ethics training that fosters one's moral sensitivity, reasoning, and discernment.

The A.B.I.D.E. and G.R.A.C.E. Models of Cultivating Compassion

Here, I share two powerful models for cultivating compassion developed by Roshi Joan Halifax. I have personally found them to be extremely useful and practical in many aspects of my life, whether personally or professionally as a physician, chaplain, and educator. For other compassion-based interventions, please read the excellent review by Kirby.[6]

The A.B.I.D.E. Model

Compassion is made up of many non-compassion elements, including attention, prosocial feelings, altruistic intention, insight, and embodiment. To capture the components that comprise compassion, the interactive processes that prime compassion, and the elements that optimize and sustain compassion, Roshi Joan Halifax formulates a heuristic model of enactive compassion called the *A.B.I.D.E. model* (Figure 7.1).[4,7] It consists of three interrelated axes: attentional and

THE A.B.I.D.E. MODEL

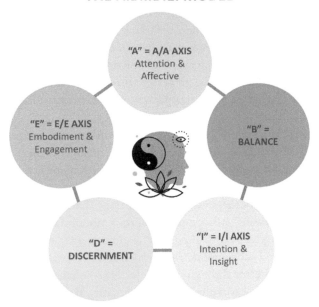

Figure 7.1 The A.B.I.D.E. model of enactive compassion.[4,7]

affective balance (the A/A axis), intention and insight (the I/I axis), and embodied and engaged processes (the E/E axis). The first two letters of the A.B.I.D.E. model stand for the A/A axis which primes mental balance. It consists of two domains: attentional and affective. The *attentional domain* involves training in attentional stability through grounding to enhance recognition of suffering. It also involves training in interoceptivity through attunement to one's own physical processes, as well as attunement to the somatic and affective states of others. As discussed previously in Chapter 5, attentional stability and interoceptivity can be developed and strengthened through mindfulness practice. The *affective domain,* the second of the A/A axis, includes cultivation of prosociality, positive regard for others, and kindness to promote enactive compassion.

The "I" and "D" in the A.B.I.D.E. model denote the I/I axis—the cognitive domains of intention and insight that prime discernment.

The first domain—*intention*—highlights the importance of setting intention to transform the suffering of others as well as oneself. Intention is primed by moral grounding—including moral imperative in how we relate to the world and moral sensitivity to discern moral issues—that defines one's moral character. The second domain—*insight*—primes a number of critical cognitive processes. These processes include metacognition that nurtures mental pliancy, self-awareness that supports reappraisal and down-regulation, perspective-taking (cognitive attunement) that allows one to understand the experience of another, and self–other distinction that preserves autonomy. Understanding impermanence, interconnectedness, happiness, and nonattachment to outcome are also included in the insight domain.

The last letter of the model stands for the E/E axis which refers to somatic dimensions. It is comprised of the embodiment and engaged domains that give rise to three key features: *ethike* (moral virtue), equanimity, and eudaemonia. The *embodiment domain* is the felt sense of another's suffering through intersubjective resonance to experience interoceptivity that is critical to prime empathy. It also allows for development of a sense of groundedness that leads to equanimity. The *engaged domain* is the experience of the body having a dispositional readiness to act in an ethical way in the world, which results in *eudaemonia*, a sense of human flourishing.[4,7]

The G.R.A.C.E. Model

To facilitate the application of the principles set forth by the A.B.I.D.E. model, especially for healthcare workers, Roshi Joan Halifax further creates the G.R.A.C.E. model of compassion-based interactions (Box 7.1).[2,8] In this model, "G" stands for *Gathering our attention*, which serves as a cue for us to pause, allowing ourselves time to get grounded. We might focus our attention on the breath, the soles of the feet on the floor, or the hands as they rest on our lap. "R" denotes *Recalling our intention* by remembering our commitment to serve others with integrity and to open our heart to the world. "A" represents *Attuning to self and other*. During self-attunement, we become familiar with our thoughts, emotions, and physical sensations.

Box 7.1 The G.R.A.C.E. model of compassion-based interactions.[2,8]

- G = Gather attention
- R = Recall intention
- A = Attune to self and other
- C = Consider what will serve
- E = Engage and End

This process of attunement and reappraisal primes the neural circuitry that regulates our emotions to bring about a healthy empathic concern. Following self-attunement, we attune to others, sensing into their experience without attachment or judgment. It is also a time when we ready ourselves for compassionate response as we attune physically (somatic empathy), emotionally (affective empathy), and cognitively (perspective-taking) to those we intend to serve. "C" stands for *Considering what will serve* by asking ourselves the following questions: What is the person in front of me hoping for? To what extent does this person trust me? What might serve this person? What am I hoping for? What am I afraid of? What might be a good outcome? What insights emerge? As Roshi Joan Halifax puts it: "This process requires attentional and affective balance, a deep sense of moral grounding, recognition of our own biases, humility, and attunement into the experience and needs of the person who is suffering."[2] "E" denotes *Engaging and Ending*. With wise discernment, we ethically engage and act. Compassionate action emerges from our acumen, openness, and connectedness. Our action might be a nod, a suggestion, a question, and sometimes "non-doing." Then, when the time is appropriate, we end and bring our interaction to a close, so that we can move on to the next moment, task, or person.[2] This model has been validated by a study on its impact on healthcare professionals.[7]

What does G.R.A.C.E. look like in practice? Personally, I found it to be a simple yet highly effective mnemonic that is easy to remember, even when I am under stress or time pressure. I can use it anywhere, whether it be an encounter with a patient, a colleague, a trainee, a hospice client, or a prisoner, or whether I am interacting with family, friends, or even people with whom I have difficulties. For example, at work, before I enter the examining room, I make use of the "threshold moment" of sanitizing my hands to gather my attention by focusing on my breath or the sensation of my hands (the "G" of G.R.A.C.E.). This simple act allows me to clear my mind, ground myself in the present, and stay open to whatever arises with curiosity. I then ask: Why I am here? Why am I really here? Really, why am I here? By asking myself this same question repeatedly, it allows me to recall my intention: to serve in whatever way I can with the immediate task at hand (the "R" of G.R.A.C.E.). It also helps me to touch deeper into the reasons of my being in the world: to heal, to alleviate suffering, and to transform. As I begin to interact with my patients, I spend some initial time listening fully to what they have to say rather than starting automatically to analyze, make a diagnosis, or formulate a treatment plan. I do this by attuning to my body, heart, and mind, noticing the sensations of my feet on the floor or my hips supported by the chair, as well as any emotions (distress, annoyance, anxiety, joy, ease) or thoughts (planning, questions, distractions) that arise. At the same time, I pay close attention to my patients, looking for any emotional cues from their tone of voice, bodily gesture, and facial expression (the "A" of G.R.A.C.E.). I consider this attunement process a kind of mutual acknowledgement, a reciprocal exchange, a sharing of trust. This process also primes what Dr. Ronald Epstein called a "shared mind"—"an intersubjective experience when ideas, intuitions, and decisions emerge not only from individuals but from the interaction among them."[9]

I then ask: What will best serve here (the "C" of G.R.A.C.E.)? How could I maintain a "strong back" of equanimity and a "soft back" of compassion[10] even in the midst of the most challenging situation? I draw on my expertise, experience, and intuition, and, at the same time, I am willing to be open, ready to see things from different perspectives, always keeping my intention in the back of my mind. I might offer a diagnosis or recommendation, and, when dealing with complex cases, I remain mindful not to indulge in an illusion of certainty (the "E" or "engaging" part of G.R.A.C.E.). I might converse with patients about their values, goals, and preferences, so that they can exercise their autonomy. Or I might remain silent, which may last only a few seconds, but it creates a sense of spaciousness, allowing a shared understanding and a deeper emotional tone to emerge. I also remind myself that sometimes, the most compassionate action is non-action, especially in situation when no medicine or surgery can cure the patient's disease, trusting that my wholehearted presence is all that is needed at that moment. I also make sure that, throughout the whole process, because I work in a pediatric setting, I do not only address the parents, but I also do the same for my patients in an age-appropriate manner (being playful, using humour, and expressing a genuine curiosity to find out what their interests are, their aspirations, and their unique concerns from a child/adolescent's perspective). Finally, as we come to the end of the visit, I make eye contact with the patients and their parents one more time, acknowledging what has transpired, and explicitly recognizing internally that the encounter is complete before I move on to the next patient (the "E" or "ending" part of G.R.A.C.E.). I must say it sounds like a lot when describing this sequence, and yes, at the beginning, we might need to recall each step deliberately. However, as we become more and more familiar with G.R.A.C.E., it will become our second nature, flowing effortlessly and spontaneously.

Inner Compassion and Its Benefits

Compassion is essential to humanity yet, for some, especially for those who work in healthcare, having compassion toward oneself may be difficult. We may castigate ourselves for our shortcomings, with our inner voice being our own harshest critic. We may reprimand ourselves bitterly for feeling angry, jealous, and contemptuous, but that only leads to self-hatred. We may also feel shame—a self-conscious emotion that arises from negative core beliefs including inadequacy, unworthiness, dishonour, regret, guilt, or disconnection. Indeed, any emotion (e.g., fear, anger, grief) that will not go away usually has an element of shame lurking behind and sustaining it. The lack of inner compassion explains partly the triad of emotional exhaustion, depersonalization, and low personal accomplishment that characterizes the burnout that is widespread in healthcare workers. Unfortunately, "self-compassion" has almost become a cliché in our society. For some, it connotes self-pity, selfishness, self-indulgence, or demotivation. Our current culture doesn't help either, as many equate "self-compassion" with weakness, self-absorption, narcissism, bypassing, or ego-centredness. To circumvent these often unconscious personal and cultural biases, "inner compassion" may be a better term as it conveys an inwardly oriented, friendly, nonjudgmental attitude that accepts one's own basic goodness without reinforcing an erroneous sense of a fixed, unchanging self.

So, what is inner compassion? It is the ability to turn understanding, acceptance, and love inward toward oneself. Rather than being self-critical, we could express self-kindness inwardly and acknowledge that shame is an innocent emotion. Instead of feeling isolated, we could recognize our common humanity as we face our weaknesses, flaws, and limitations, as well as accepting that shame is a universal emotion.[11] Not ruminating about past events, upsets, or failures, we could plant ourselves firmly in the present with mindfulness. If we truly aspire to serve the world with compassion, we need to first cultivate kindness toward ourselves. As the 14th Dalai Lama said: "For someone to develop genuine compassion towards others, first he or she must have a basis upon which to cultivate compassion, and that basis is the ability to connect to one's own feelings and to care for one's own welfare. . . . Caring for others requires caring for oneself."

This is supported by numerous studies showing that inner compassion is crucial for well-being.[12] Higher levels of optimism, life satisfaction, happiness, perceived competence, and motivation are found in people who are compassionate toward themselves.[13-17] Inner compassion is also associated with lower levels of self-criticism, depression, anxiety, stress, rumination, body shame, perfectionism, and fear of failure.[18-25] The protective effects of inner compassion against these negative states of mind may result from better physiological responses to stress, as indicated by decreased plasma concentrations of cortisol and interleukin-6 and increased heart-rate variability (vagal tone), as well as better blood glucose control in diabetes.[26-30] Importantly, inner compassion is linked to more personal initiative, curiosity, intellectual flexibility, emotional intelligence, wisdom, and self-determination, as well as to feelings of social connectedness and autonomy—qualities that are essential for a meaningful and flourishing life.[13,31-33]

Specific to healthcare workers, inner compassion improves professional quality of life and is protective against empathy fatigue and burnout.[34-36] Over the years, in my experience as a teacher in a mindfulness and compassion training course for healthcare workers, a crucial turning point occurs when participants became aware of a lack of inner compassion as well as the shame and guilt hidden behind it. This is often a pivotal juncture where many begin to realize how much these negative states have contributed to their emotional exhaustion and burnout. From there, a strong determination arises in them to embark on a journey of healing and well-being through the deliberate cultivation of mindfulness and compassion.

Given its many benefits, what are some ways to build inner compassion? I will offer some strategies here based on Dr. Paul Gilbert's compassion-focused therapy, an extension and adjunct to behavioural cognitive therapy.[37-42] As discussed in Chapter 6, a lack of inner compassion usually arises from a self-critical cycle which activates and perpetuates the threat system while it suppresses the affiliative system. The key, then, is to shift this dynamic in favour of the affiliative system (Figure 7.2). Mindfulness training is particularly valuable because it helps to increase our awareness of our own suffering as well as our self-critical responses that may include somatic sensations, emotions, and behaviours. With increased awareness, we are in a better position to choose to respond differently. For example, we could choose intentionally to dampen our self-critical responses by breathing slowly and deeply into the belly. This is a very effective and readily available means to calm the body and mind by tapping into our parasympathetic nervous system. Mindfulness also helps us to attain attention stability, so that when our mind wanders or when it leaps back to self-critical thinking, we can deliberately redirect our attention back to the breath to remain calm. By activating the affiliative system, we are better able to *think* in more compassionate ways (e.g., reminding ourselves that no one is perfect, that shame is a universal emotion, and that "pain is inevitable but suffering is optional"). We could cultivate compassionate thoughts and feelings further by engaging in activities such as writing letters to ourselves or keeping a thought diary when we are struggling with something in particular, by recalling a benefactor or someone (even a pet) who cares about us deeply (see Chapter 3), or by

THE INNER COMPASSION (VIRTUOUS) CYCLE

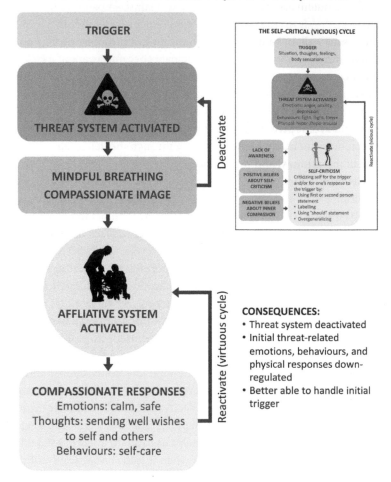

Figure 7.2 The inner compassion cycle that activates the affiliative system and deactivates the threat system. Inset shows the self-critical cycle (Figure 6.2) for compassion. Adapted from Saulsman et al.[42]

remembering what we are grateful for in our daily lives. Activating the affiliative system also allows us to be in a better position to *behave* and take care of ourselves in more compassionate ways: for example, we can go for a walk in nature, spend some time in solitude, or listen to our favourite music.

Drawing from my own personal experience, as we build inner compassion with patience and diligence, we gradually develop a sense of stability, clarity, and deep inner strength. Instead of being overwhelmed or pushing away our suffering, our flaws, or our shame, we can befriend them, knowing that they are part and parcel of being human. By acknowledging our own pain, we can begin to appreciate the depths of other's suffering, which opens up a gateway in our quest for insights and wisdom. In the process, we begin to heal, transform, and experience an interior movement so that when we serve, it comes from a much deeper place that is beyond our personalities, needs, fears, or compulsions. As we become more at ease with life's challenges, ambiguity, and uncertainty, genuine compassion toward self and others emerges that is spontaneous, unconditional, and free of expectations of any preconceived outcomes.

Last, I would like to share with you a passage by Charles Eisenstein that I found to be particularly insightful:

> Do not tell yourself that you shouldn't be judgmental. . . . That's because judgmentality withers away of its own accord when compassion arises, and compassion arises, naturally and effortlessly, from the sober, unsentimental understanding of the origin of a person's behavior. . . . Compassion for others and, even more, for oneself, doesn't require overlooking flaws or ignoring the shadow side. Innate divinity does not lie apart from our most shameful sins—it lies within them. Underneath everything you are and everything you do is a sweet, innocent being, doing its best to cope with the confusing world into which it has wandered. You are a pure, earnest child plunged into a maelstrom with only the most exiguous of threads connecting you back to your Mother. Do not judge yourself too harshly, for you have done your best with the knowledge available to you. When you can understand every action, of yourself and others, as the touchingly naive response of an innocent

baby-in-an-adult-body to a world gone incomprehensibly wrong; seeking, as all creatures will, to avoid pain in a very painful world; buffeted, like milkweed in a storm, by environmental forces vastly dwarfing the power of any single individual; concealing a fathomless well of loss and private sadness; taking on a measure of difficulty and suffering at the very edge of one's capacity; and yet, heroically, striving, surviving, and transcending circumstances beyond any reasonable expectation; then you will see glory in every person, a divine and radiant beauty.[43]

Compassionate Leadership to Build a Compassionate Culture

While contemplative practices and inner compassion focus primarily on the personal level, equally important is compassionate leadership at the system level if we are to bring about a compassionate culture. Culture is the combination of "values and beliefs that characterize organizations as transmitted by the socialization experiences that newcomers have, the decisions made by management, and the stories and myths people tell and retell about their organizations."[44] Research has shown that leadership plays the most powerful role in transmitting the core values and beliefs of organizations.[45] Leadership can be conceptualized as "a process whereby intentional influence is exerted over other people to guide, structure, and facilitate activities and relationships in a group or organization."[46] From this definition, we can distinguish between leader and leadership. *Leader* is a specialized role that an individual occupies, whereas *leadership* is a process of influence—anyone in a group or organization may exercise leadership at any point. The complex interactions between people and situations will affect the emergence of compassion. In other words, compassion is also a characteristic of interactions rather than necessarily of individuals. In what follows, I will first describe the characteristics of compassionate leaders, especially in those who hold formal leadership positions. I will then discuss the influence process perspective of leadership in which informal collective leadership can bring about and reinforce a compassionate culture.

Compassionate leadership in an organizational context can be understood as having four components: attending, understanding, empathizing, and helping.[47] According to this model, the first task for leaders is to *attend* to those they lead by devoting adequate time to listen deeply and to develop an appreciation of the challenges their staff face. The second task is to appraise and *understand* the causes of distress for one's staff. While these first two tasks may seem obvious for leadership, in high-stress situations and under time constraints, staff often feel they are not listened to and that their leaders do not understand the situations they face.[48] These two tasks—attending and understanding—therefore, cannot be overemphasized. The third task for leaders is empathizing, which is linked to emotion and perspective-taking. Compassionate leaders are emotionally in touch with, able to endure, and yet not overidentify with the distress of their staff. The fourth task is helping, which has four elements: scope, the range of resources available; scale, the volume of resources offered; speed, the timeliness of the response; and specialization, the extent to which the response meets the real needs of the staff.[49]

These four tasks of compassionate leadership are especially relevant in healthcare. Healthcare is a vocation in which a core value of compassion is embedded among those who chose this path. Motivated by a desire to serve others, healthcare workers are highly skilled and are intent on doing a good job by meeting the highest possible standard. They require support rather than unilateral direction from leaders, enabling rather than controlling interventions, and flexibility rather than adherence to rigid rules. When leaders listen, empathize with, and understand their staff—what motivates them, what their challenges are, what assistance is needed—authentic compassionate interactions then take place. In this way, leaders reflect, embody, and amplify organizational values. Studies have shown that the stronger the alignment between organizational values and those of staff, the higher the levels of staff's commitment, engagement, and satisfaction.[50]

While a compassionate culture can be nurtured by leaders who embody compassion, compassionate leadership is not restricted to those with official titles. Informal collective leadership is equally important to create and sustain a compassionate culture. *Organizational compassion* can be cultivated when there is collective awareness and acknowledgment of the suffering within a workplace that values such awareness.[50] Staff can collectively feel and express their concerns through narratives and communication to share freely their observations, thoughts, and emotions. As a result of increasing awareness and communication, collective helping can then emerge within an organization where the sufferings are legitimized and resourced for. Beyond its impact on individuals, compassion also has the potential to radiate out, so that those receiving compassion are better able to care for others,[49] replenish the emotional resources they need, and protect against burnout.[49,51] The positive ripple effects of compassion can also spread to others beyond patients and caregivers, inspiring others to act for the common good.[49,51] The theory of *positivity resonance* explains how moments of interpersonal compassion benefit people through a natural synchronization of bodies and minds that enhances health and well-being.[52]

The need for compassionate leadership is not confined within an organization. Health and social care services must be coordinated in order to meet the needs of patients, service users, and communities.[52] This integrated approach requires leaders to work together at a wider system level that crosses the boundaries between organizations, governmental agencies, and regulatory bodies.

What does compassionate leadership look like in practice? In addition to the preceding description, I found that the work of Dr. John Paul Lederach,[53] a leading conflict transformation expert, also applies to compassionate leadership. In my view, it is critical for compassionate leaders to articulate clearly their vision, help staff make meaning, promote collective awareness, cultivate a non-anxious presence, focus on process and dynamics, and take a long-term view. For example, as a physician-leader, I make it clear that my vision is not only to provide the best care to patients through clinical service, research, and education, but also to foster a multidisciplinary, collaborative, and respectful team environment so that each team member enjoys opportunities for educational advancement, work satisfaction, and personal growth. I invite my staff to envision what a truly caring and compassionate culture looks like, not only for patients and their families, but also for each other as co-workers. I help my staff make meaning of their work by asking them regularly to recall the reasons why they chose to work in healthcare and what their deep intention is to work in a children's hospital. I encourage them to express their observations, concerns, and feelings through narratives and communications with others to build collective awareness. I endeavour to cultivate a non-anxious presence by being present with a sense of openness, peace, and nonjudgment, interacting with my staff mindfully, empathically, and nonviolently.[54,55] When conflicts occur, I choose consciously to defocus on people, problems, and crises, and instead focus on patterns, emotional processes, and relational dynamics. I resist the tendency to blame or point fingers, and I watch for relational patterns such as unspoken rules in the system and the drama triangle of victim, rescuer, and persecutor,[56] as well as in- and out-group dynamics. Last, I remind myself that complex problems do not arise in a linear fashion and hence they cannot be solved with a linear solution. I remain cognizant that changes in a complex system can take a long time, and that the desired outcomes may not come to fruition during my tenure. While this fact is not always easy to accept, nevertheless, I initiate change by encouraging and reminding myself that someone needs to take the first step.

System Changes for Compassionate Healthcare

While cultivating compassion at the individual level and promoting compassionate leadership are essential, they are not sufficient to return healthcare to its compassionate core. Organizations and systems must make commitments that enable rather than impede compassionate, high-quality healthcare. Inputs from patients, family members, healthcare professionals, educators, administrators, health policymakers, measurement experts, and researchers must be obtained, synthesized, and enacted to create a more compassionate healthcare system. It is worth noting that in a climate where cost and access have often been cited as key priorities among patients and healthcare providers, in a recent survey, 85% of patients reported compassion as a very important factor, whereas only 31% cited cost and 48% considered wait time as being very important to them.[57]

Dr. Beth Lown, Associate Professor of Medicine at Harvard Medical School, representing a working meeting among these stakeholders, reported seven commitments that organizations and systems must adopt and take action on if they are to embed compassionate care in all aspects of training, research, patient care, and organizational life. They include (1) *commitment to compassionate healthcare leadership*—leaders share, disseminate, implement, and assess exemplary compassionate care leadership practices, tools, and quality standards; (2) *commitment to teach compassion*—educators integrate, teach, and assess the knowledge, skills, and attitudes required for health professional students, trainees, and practising clinicians to provide compassionate care; (3) *commitment to value and reward compassion*—stakeholders ensure that healthcare institutions value, support, and reward the cognitive, emotional, and collaborative work and time required for caregivers to provide compassionate care; (4) *commitment to support caregivers*—leaders and systems support the wellness and resilience of healthcare professionals and address systemic factors that contribute to burnout; (5) *commitment to partner with patients and families*—leaders and organizations invite patients and families to participate in and co-create processes and policies that promote compassionate care; (6) *commitment to build compassion into healthcare delivery*—healthcare organizations, systems, and policymakers prioritize opportunities and time for personal interactions and continuity of shared information and relationships; and (7) *commitment to deepening our understanding of compassion*—researchers articulate and stakeholders measure the characteristics and outcomes of compassionate healthcare at all levels (individuals, teams, groups, and organizations).[58]

In addition to the institutional level, broader discussions about overall priorities and policy decisions must also be conducted at the societal level. With compassion as a fundamental principle, these discussions are instrumental in guiding decisions on the allocation of scarce resources to meet other social needs in addition to healthcare.

Benefits of Compassion in Healthcare

What are the benefits of compassion in healthcare? Numerous studies have shown that compassion is critical to improve patient outcomes ranging from physiological and psychological health to better self-care behaviours. Compassion also benefits the caregivers by serving as an antidote to burnout. From a system perspective, compassion improves healthcare quality, increases revenue, and reduces costs. In what follows, I will review the benefits of compassion to patients, caregivers, and the healthcare system. For an excellent systematic review, please refer to Drs. Stephen Trzeciak and Anthony Mazzarelli's book *Compassionomics*.[59]

Physiological Benefits of Compassion to Patients

There is ample research evidence showing that compassion improves patient outcomes at a physiological level. For example, patients undergoing surgery were calmer, required less anesthesia during surgery, reported less pain postoperatively, and exhibited better wound healing when they experienced compassionate care from doctors and nurses.[60–62] Patients also recovered faster after heart attack, with reduced hospitalization, and they had better outcomes after major trauma.[62,63] Similarly, those who suffered from chronic pain, including back pain, migraine headache, and abdominal pain from irritable bowel syndrome, reported less symptoms with decreased pain intensity, frequency, and functional impairment.[64–66] Patients with diabetes had better blood glucose control and reduced serious complications such as ketoacidosis and coma.[67,68] Interestingly, even patients with common cold fared better when their doctors were empathic; the duration and severity of their symptoms were reduced as a result of better immunity from increased immune cytokine interleukin-8.[69] Importantly, compassion that involved both verbal communication and nonverbal body language (e.g., making direct eye contact, smiling, nodding, and leaning in toward the patient) also led to better patient physical, cognitive, and psychological functioning.[70]

Psychological Benefits of Compassion to Patients

Compassion-based interventions are highly effective in treating depression, anxiety, eating disorders, psychotic disorders, and posttraumatic stress disorder, as well as suicidal ideation.[71-80] These interventions exert their effects partly through decreased patient self-criticism and shame and increased inner compassion.[80,81] The therapeutic alliance also plays a role. Therapists who were compassionate helped reduce symptoms by ameliorating their patients' feelings of hopelessness[82-84] and increasing patient compliance.[85] Interestingly, perceived compassion by nursing home residents, but not by the caregivers, was associated with lower depression symptoms.[86] This is important because it indicates that appraisal of our own compassion may not match what patients actually experience.

In addition to mental health disorders, compassion alleviates psychological distress related to physical illness. Physician empathy was associated with greater patient satisfaction, increased self-efficacy, reduced emotional distress, and less anxiety in patients with cancer.[87-89] Clinicians who were compassionate when breaking bad news reduced patient anxiety, uncertainty, and physiological arousal.[90-93] Interestingly, compassion is cumulative: the number of empathic responses from physicians correlated with declines in patient anxiety.[94] These effects likely result from better psychological adjustment to cancer diagnosis leading to improved psychological quality of life.[88,95-99] Similarly, patients experienced lower emotional distress in primary care settings when clinicians showed compassion.[100-102] Importantly, patients who received compassionate clinician communication about high recovery expectations had better clinical outcomes than those who received low expectations.[93,103,104] Finally, compassion motivates patient self-care and adherence to therapy through increased patient engagement, enablement, and trust, which leads to better long-term outcomes and enhanced quality of life.[105-115]

Compassion as an Antidote to Burnout
for Healthcare Professionals

Research has suggested an inverse relationship between compassion and burnout; that is, high compassion is protective against burnout, whereas low compassion increases the risk of burnout.[116] For example, higher compassion in medical trainees and practising physicians is linked to decreased depression symptoms and an increased sense of personal accomplishment, as well as to enhanced resilience and quality of life.[117-121] The same holds true for nurses.[122,123] Encouragingly, mindfulness and compassion training reduces physician symptoms of burnout and depression and improves their sense of well-being.[124,125] A culture of compassion is also important: there is less emotional exhaustion and better psychological vitality among these healthcare workers.[126,127] Importantly, a compassionate workplace culture creates a virtuous cycle. Empathic care improves patient experience, which in turn transforms the caregiver experience in a meaningful way, allowing caregivers to build personal resilience against burnout.[126,128-132] Compassion not only benefits frontline workers, it also enhances the resilience of physician leaders and administrators in healthcare organizations.[133,134] Last, as discussed earlier in this chapter, inner compassion improves the quality of life of caregivers and is a powerful protector against empathy fatigue and burnout.[34-36]

Benefits of Compassion to the Healthcare System

From a system perspective, compassion improves healthcare quality, increases revenues, and reduces costs. It has been shown that depersonalization, emotional exhaustion, and lack of compassion can lead to major medical or surgical errors that jeopardize patient safety and quality standards.[118,135-139] These adverse events also cause emotional harms on patients, who have repeatedly emphasized emotional over physical harms.[140-143] Compassion is therefore critical to improve patient safety. It is linked to higher levels of perceived clinician competence, which in turn leads to higher quality care through a variety of potential mechanisms including[59] (1) higher levels of clinician commitment to make an extra effort to ensure best clinical outcomes; (2) higher standards of care among clinicians; (3) increased patient trust, which results in enhanced therapeutic alliance; and (4) more patient self-disclosure of pertinent health and personal information.[144-149]

Compassionate care also increases hospital revenues and reduces healthcare costs. Hospitals with a compassionate or patient-centred culture are more likely to get higher patient satisfaction ratings and are also more profitable.[150,151] Indeed, patients are willing to pay more for compassionate care.[152,153] Better patient experience not only drives revenues, it also lowers costs.[154-157] One reason is that patient-centred care curbs excessive healthcare utilization by reducing unnecessary referrals to specialists or the performance of unwarranted diagnostic tests.[158-161] Another reason is that compassionate care enhances patient compliance, thereby saving costs from preventable hospitalizations.[105-115] A compassionate culture also boosts institutional financial performance because when caregivers are less emotionally exhausted, there are less costs associated with turnover, absenteeism, or decreased productivity.[117,162-165] Last, compassion lowers malpractice costs. Several studies have indicated that doctor–patient relationship, or a lack thereof, is a major factor when patients decide to pursue malpractice litigation.[166-170]

Summary of Key Points

- Important preliminaries to foster compassion include taking care of one's basic needs (having enough sleep, a balanced diet, regular exercise), cultivating nourishing relationships, and learning to pause (by focusing on the breath or the sensation of the feet on the floor).
- Contemplative traditions offer many time-tested and skilful approaches for the cultivation of compassion, resilience, and equanimity. These skills include awareness practices that help one recognize somatic responses and emotional arousal; mindfulness

practices that stabilize attention, monitor thoughts, and regulate emotions; insight practices that develop one's capacity to pause, listen, inquire, explore, and reflect with openness and curiosity; compassion training that primes kindness, generosity, patience, gratitude, and other prosocial attributes; and ethics training that fosters one's moral sensitivity, reasoning, and discernment.

- The A.B.I.D.E. model of enactive compassion consists of three interrelated axes: attention and affective domains that prime mental balance (the A/A axis), intention and insight domains that lead to discernment (the I/I axis), and embodied and engaged domains that result in moral virtue, equanimity, and eudaemonia/flourishing (the E/E axis).

- The G.R.A.C.E. model of compassion-based interactions consists of five components: gathering attention, recalling intention, attuning to self and other, considering what will serve, and engaging/ending.

- To build inner compassion, we need to shift from the threat system to activate the affiliative system. By intentionally slowing down, mindfulness training is particularly valuable in allowing us to choose to respond differently. By activating the affiliative system, we are better able to *think* and *behave* in more compassionate ways.

- Leader is a specialized role that an individual occupies. Compassionate leadership has four components: attending, understanding, empathizing, and helping. When leaders listen, empathize with, understand, and help their staff, authentic compassionate interactions take place. In this way, leaders reflect, embody, and amplify organizational values.

- Leadership is not only a formal role, it is also a process of influence—anyone in a group or organization may exercise leadership at any point. Organizational compassion can be cultivated when there is collective awareness, acknowledgement, and communication of the sufferings within a workplace so that the sufferings are legitimized and resourced for to allow compassionate exchanges to emerge. Each of us can be a leader to foster compassion in whatever spheres we are in: personal, workplace, community, system, and planet.

- To create a more compassionate healthcare system, inputs from patients, family members, healthcare professionals, educators, administrators, health policymakers, measurement experts, and researchers must be obtained, synthesized, and enacted.
- Compassion is critical to improve patient outcomes ranging from physiological and psychological health to better self-care behaviours. Compassion also benefits the caregivers by serving as an antidote to burnout. From a healthcare system perspective, compassion improves quality, increases revenue, and reduces costs.

References

1. Dąbrowski K. The theory of positive disintegration. *Int J Psychiatry.* 1966;2:229–244.
2. Halifax J. *Standing at the Edge.* New York: Martin's Press; 2018.
3. Frankl V. Alleged quote. Viktor Frankl Institut; 2020. https://www.univie.ac.at/logotherapy/quote_stimulus.html
4. Halifax J. A heuristic model of enactive compassion. *Curr Opin Support Palliat Care.* 2012;6(2):228–235.
5. Rushton CH, Kaszniak AW, Halifax JS. Addressing moral distress: Application of a framework to palliative care practice. *J Palliat Med.* 2013;16(9):1080–1088.
6. Kirby JN. Compassion interventions: The programmes, the evidence, and implications for research and practice. *Psychol Psychother.* 2017;90(3):432–455.
7. Rushton CH, Sellers DE, Heller KS, Spring B, Dossey BM, Halifax J. Impact of a contemplative end-of-life training program: Being with dying. *Palliat Support Care.* 2009;7(4):405–414.
8. Halifax J. G.R.A.C.E. for nurses: Cultivating compassion in nurse/patient interactions. *J Nurse Educ Pract.* 2014;4(1):121–128.
9. Epstein R. *Attending: Medicine, Mindfulness, and Humanity.* New York: Scribner; 2017.
10. Rushton CH, Kaszniak AW, Halifax JS. A framework for understanding moral distress among palliative care clinicians. *J Palliat Med.* 2013;16(9):1074–1079.
11. Neff K. *Self-Compassion: The Proven Power of Being Kind to Yourself.* New York: William Morrow; 2015.

12. Neff K, Germer C. Self-compassion and psychological well-being. In: Seppälä EM, Simon-Thomas E, Brown SL, Worline MC, Cameron CD, Doty JR, eds. *The Oxford Handbook of Compassion Science.* New York: Oxford University Press; 2017:371–386.

13. Neff KD, Rude SS, Kirkpatrick K. An examination of self-compassion in relation to positive psychological functioning and personality traits. *J Res Pers.* 2007;41:908–916.

14. Neff KD, Pisitsungkagarn K, Hseih Y. Self-compassion and self-construal in the United States, Thailand, and Taiwan. *J Cross Cult Psychol.* 2008;39:267–285.

15. Neff KD, Hseih Y, Dejitthirat K. Self-compassion, achievement goals, and coping with academic failure. *Self Identity.* 2005;4:263–287.

16. Hollis-Walker L, Colosimo K. Mindfulness, self-compassion, and happiness in non-meditators: A theoretical and empirical examination. *Pers Individ Differ.* 2011;50:222–227.

17. Zessin U, Dickhauser O, Garbade S. The relationship between self-compassion and well-being: A meta-analysis. *Appl Psychol Health Well Being.* 2015;7(3):340–364.

18. Smeets E, Neff K, Alberts H, Peters M. Meeting suffering with kindness: Effects of a brief self-compassion intervention for female college students. *J Clin Psychol.* 2014;70(9):794–807.

19. Shapira LB, Mongrain M. The benefits of self-compassion and optimism exercises for individuals vulnerable to depression. *J Posit Psychol.* 2010;5:377–389.

20. Neff KD, Germer CK. A pilot study and randomized controlled trial of the mindful self-compassion program. *J Clin Psychol.* 2013;69(1):28–44.

21. Albertson ER, Neff KD, Dill-Shackleford KE. Self-compassion and body dissatisfaction in women: A randomized controlled trial of a brief meditation intervention. *Mindfulness.* 2014;6:444–454.

22. Raes F. Rumination and worry as mediators of the relationship between self-compassion and depression and anxiety. *Pers Individ Differ.* 2010;48:757–761.

23. Finlay-Jones AL, Rees CS, Kane RT. Self-compassion, emotion regulation and stress among Australian psychologists: Testing an emotion regulation model of self-compassion using structural equation modeling. *PLoS One.* 2015;10(7):e0133481.

24. Daye CA, Webb JB, Jafari N. Exploring self-compassion as a refuge against recalling the body-related shaming of caregiver eating messages on dimensions of objectified body consciousness in college women. *Body Image.* 2014;11:547–556.

25. Blatt SJ. Representational structures in psychopathology. In: Cicchetti D, Toth S, eds. *Rochester Symposium on Developmental Psychopathology:*

Emotion, Cognition, and Representation. Vol 6. Rochester: University of Rochester Press; 1995:1–34.

26. Rockliff H, Gilbert P, McEwan K, Lightman S, Glover D. A pilot exploration of heart rate variability and salivary cortisol responses to compassion-focused imagery. *Clin Neuropsychiatry.* 2008;5:132–139.

27. Arch JJ, Brown KW, Dean DJ, Landy LN, Brown KD, Laudenslager ML. Self-compassion training modulates alpha-amylase, heart rate variability, and subjective responses to social evaluative threat in women. *Psychoneuroendocrinology.* 2014;42:49–58.

28. Friis AM, Johnson MH, Cutfield RG, Consedine NS. Does kindness matter? Self-compassion buffers the negative impact of diabetes-distress on HbA1c. *Diabet Med.* 2015;32(12):1634–1640.

29. Breines J, Toole A, Tu C, Chen S. Self-compassion, body image, and self-reported disordered eating. *Self Identity.* 2014;13:432–448.

30. Breines JG, Thoma MV, Gianferante D, Hanlin L, Chen X, Rohleder N. Self-compassion as a predictor of interleukin-6 response to acute psychosocial stress. *Brain Behav Immun.* 2014;37:109–114.

31. Heffernan M, Quinn Griffin MT, Sister Rita M, Fitzpatrick JJ. Self-compassion and emotional intelligence in nurses. *Int J Nurs Pract.* 2010;16(4):366–373.

32. Martin MM, Staggers SM, Anderson CM. The relationships between cognitive flexibility with dogmatism, intellectual flexibility, preference for consistency, and self-compassion. *Commun Res Rep.* 2011;28:275–280.

33. Magnus CMR, Kowalski KC, McHugh TLF. The role of self-compassion in women's self-determined motives to exercise and exercise-related outcomes. *Self Identity.* 2010;9:363–382.

34. Raab K, Sogge K, Parker N, Flament MF. Mindfulness-based stress reduction and self-compassion among mental healthcare professionals: A pilot study. *Ment Health Relig Cult.* 2015;18:503–512.

35. Montero-Marin J, Zubiaga F, Cereceda M, Piva Demarzo MM, Trenc P, Garcia-Campayo J. Burnout subtypes and absence of self-compassion in primary healthcare professionals: A cross-sectional study. *PLoS One.* 2016;11(6):e0157499.

36. Duarte J, Pinto-Gouveia J, Cruz B. Relationships between nurses' empathy, self-compassion and dimensions of professional quality of life: A cross-sectional study. *Int J Nurs Stud.* 2016;60:1–11.

37. Gilbert P. *The Compassionate Mind.* London: Constable & Robinson; 2009.

38. Gilbert P. *Compassion Focused Therapy: Distinctive Features.* East Sussex, UK: Routledge; 2010.

39. Gilbert P, Irons C. Focused therapies and compassionate mind training for shame and self-attacking. In: Gilbert P, ed. *Compassion: Conceptualisations, Research and Use in Psychotherapy.* New York: Routledge; 2005:263–325.

40. Gilbert P, Procter S. Compassionate mind training for people with high shame and self-criticism: Overview and pilot study. *Clin Psychol Psychother.* 2006;13:353–379.

41. Gilbert P. The origins and nature of compassion focused therapy. *Br J Clin Psychol.* 2014;53(1):6–41.

42. Saulsman L, Campbell B, Sng A. Building self-compassion: From self-criticism to self-kindness. Perth, Western Australia Centre for Clinical Interventions; 2017: https://www.cci.health.wa.gov.au/Resources/Looking-After-Yourself/Self-Compassion

43. Eisenstein C. *The Yoga of Eating: Transcending Diets and Dogma to Nourish the Natural Self.* Washington, DC: NewTrends Publishing; 2003.

44. Schneider B, Barbera KM, eds. *The Oxford Handbook of Organisational Climate and Culture.* Oxford: Oxford University Press; 2014.

45. Schneider B, Gonzalez-Roma V, Ostroff C, West MA. Organizational climate and culture: Reflections on the history of the constructs in the Journal of Applied Psychology. *J Appl Psychol.* 2017;102(3):468–482.

46. Yukl S. *Leadership in Organisations* (8th ed.). Harlow, UK: Pearson Education Limited; 2013.

47. Atkins PWB, Parker SK. Understanding individual compassion in organisations: The role of appraisals and psychological flexibility. *Acad Manage Rev.* 2012;37(4):524–546.

48. National Health Service. NHS Staff Management and Health Service Quality. Results from the NHS Staff Survey and Related Data. Report to the Department of Health. 2011. http://www.dh.gov.uk/health/2011/08/nhs-staff-management/

49. Lilius JM, Kanov J, Dutton JE, Worline MC, Maitlis S. Compassion revealed: What we know about compassion at work (and where we need to know more). In: Cameron K, Spreitzer G, eds. *The Oxford Handbook of Positive Organisational Scholarship.* New York: Oxford University Press; 2011:273–288.

50. West MA, Chowla R. Compassionate leadership for compassionate health care. In: Gilbert P, ed. *Compassion: Concepts, Research and Applications.* New York: Routledge; 2017:237–257.

51. Dutton JE, Workman KM, Hardin AE. Compassion at work. *Annu Rev Organ Psychol Organ Behav.* 2014;1(1):277–304.

52. Fredrickson B. *Love 2.0: How Our Supreme Emotion Affects Everything We Feel, Think, Do, and Become.* New York: Hudson Street Press; 2013.

53. Lederach JP. *The Little Book of Conflict Transformation.* New York: Good Books; 2014.

54. Rosenberg MB. *Nonviolent Communication: A Language of Life.* Encinitas, CA: PuddleDancer Press; 2003.

55. Sofer OJ. *Say What You Mean: A Mindful Approach to Nonviolent Communication.* Boulder, CO: Shambhala Publications; 2018.

56. Karpman SB. *A Game Free Life. The Definitive Book on the Drama Triangle and Compassion Triangle by the Originator and Author. The New Transactional Analysis of Intimacy, Openness, and Happiness.* San Francisco, CA: Drama Triangle Publications; 2014.

57. Applied Clinical Trials. Survey reveals 85% percent of patients choose compassion over pricing when choosing a doctor. 2018. http://www.appliedclinicaltrialsonline.com/survey-reveals-85-percent-patients-choose-compassion-over-pricing-when-choosing-doctor

58. Lown BA. Seven guiding commitments: Making the US healthcare system more compassionate. *J Patient Exp.* 2014;1(2):6–15.

59. Trzeciak S, Mazzarelli A. *Compassionomics: The Revolutionary Scientific Evidence that Caring Makes a Difference.* Pensacola, FL: Studer Group, LLC; 2019.

60. Egbert LD, Battit G, Turndorf H, Beecher HK. The value of the preoperative visit by an anesthetist: A study of doctor–patient rapport. *JAMA.* 1963;185(7):553–555.

61. Egbert LD, Battit GE, Welch CE, Bartlett MK. Reduction of postoperative pain by encouragement and instruction of patients: A study of doctor-patient rapport. *N Engl J Med.* 1964;270:825–827.

62. Pereira L, Figueiredo-Braga M, Carvalho IP. Preoperative anxiety in ambulatory surgery: The impact of an empathic patient-centered approach on psychological and clinical outcomes. *Patient Educ Couns.* 2016;99(5):733–738.

63. Mumford E, Schlesinger HJ, Glass GV. The effect of psychological intervention on recovery from surgery and heart attacks: An analysis of the literature. *Am J Public Health.* 1982;72(2):141–151.

64. Dibbelt S, Schaidhammer M, Fleischer C, Greitemann B. Patient–doctor interaction in rehabilitation: The relationship between perceived interaction quality and long-term treatment results. *Patient Educ Couns.* 2009;76(3):328–335.

65. Attar HS, Chandramani S. Impact of physician empathy on migraine disability and migraineur compliance. *Ann Indian Acad Neurol.* 2012;15(Suppl 1):S89–94.

66. Kaptchuk TJ, Kelley JM, Conboy LA, et al. Components of placebo effect: Randomised controlled trial in patients with irritable bowel syndrome. *BMJ.* 2008;336(7651):999–1003.

67. Hojat M, Louis DZ, Markham FW, Wender R, Rabinowitz C, Gonnella JS. Physicians' empathy and clinical outcomes for diabetic patients. *Acad Med.* 2011;86(3):359–364.

68. Del Canale S, Louis DZ, Maio V, et al. The relationship between physician empathy and disease complications: An empirical study of primary care physicians and their diabetic patients in Parma, Italy. *Acad Med.* 2012;87(9):1243–1249.

69. Rakel DP, Hoeft TJ, Barrett BP, Chewning BA, Craig BM, Niu M. Practitioner empathy and the duration of the common cold. *Fam Med.* 2009;41(7):494–501.

70. Ambady N, Koo J, Rosenthal R, Winograd CH. Physical therapists' non-verbal communication predicts geriatric patients' health outcomes. *Psychol Aging.* 2002;17(3):443–452.

71. Judge L, Cleghorn A, McEwan K, Gilbert P. An exploration of group-based compassion focused therapy for a heterogeneous range of clients presenting to a community mental health team. *Int J Cogn Ther.* 2012;5:420–429.

72. Gilbert P, Procter S. Compassionate mind training for people with high shame and self-criticism: Overview and pilot study. *Clin Psychol Psychother.* 2006;13:353–379.

73. Graser J, Höfling V, Weßlau C, Mendes A, Stangier U. Effects of a 12-week mindfulness, compassion, and loving kindness program on chronic depression: A pilot within-subjects wait-list controlled trial. *J Cogn Psychother.* 2016;30:35–49.

74. Noorbala F, Borjali A, Ahmadian-Attari MM, Noorbala AA. Effectiveness of compassionate mind training on depression, anxiety, and self-criticism in a group of Iranian depressed patients. *Iran J Psychiatry.* 2013;8(3):113–117.

75. Johnson SB, Goodnight BL, Zhang H, Daboin I, Patterson B, Kaslow NJ. Compassion-based meditation in African Americans: Self-criticism mediates changes in depression. *Suicide Life Threat Behav.* 2018;48(2):160–168.

76. Au TM, Sauer-Zavala S, King MW, Petrocchi N, Barlow DH, Litz BT. Compassion-based therapy for trauma-related shame and posttraumatic stress: Initial evaluation using a multiple baseline design. *Behav Ther.* 2017;48(2):207–221.

77. Kelly AC, Wisniewski L, Martin-Wagar C, Hoffman E. Group-based compassion-focused therapy as an adjunct to outpatient treatment for eating disorders: A pilot randomized controlled trial. *Clin Psychol Psychother.* 2017;24(2):475–487.

78. Braehler C, Gumley A, Harper J, Wallace S, Norrie J, Gilbert P. Exploring change processes in compassion focused therapy in psychosis: Results of a feasibility randomized controlled trial. *Br J Clin Psychol.* 2013;52(2):199–214.

79. Laithwaite H, O'Hanlon M, Collins P, et al. Recovery After Psychosis (RAP): A compassion focused programme for individuals residing in high security settings. *Behav Cogn Psychother.* 2009;37(5):511–526.

80. Graser J, Stangier U. Compassion and loving-kindness meditation: An overview and prospects for the application in clinical samples. *Harv Rev Psychiatry.* 2018;26(4):201–215.

81. Kirby JN, Tellegen CL, Steindl SR. A meta-analysis of compassion-based interventions: Current state of knowledge and future directions. *Behav Ther.* 2017;48(6):778–792.

82. Ilardi SS, Craighead WE. The role of nonspecific factors in cognitive-behavior therapy for depression. *Clin Psychol (New York).* 1994;1:138–156.

83. Burns DD, Nolen-Hoeksema S. Therapeutic empathy and recovery from depression in cognitive-behavioral therapy: A structural equation model. *J Consult Clin Psychol.* 1992;60(3):441–449.

84. Blatt SJ, Quinlan DM, Zuroff DC, Pilkonis PA. Interpersonal factors in brief treatment of depression: Further analyses of the National Institute of Mental Health Treatment of Depression Collaborative Research Program. *J Consult Clin Psychol.* 1996;64(1):162–171.

85. Kaplan JE, Keeley RD, Engel M, Emsermann C, Brody D. Aspects of patient and clinician language predict adherence to antidepressant medication. *J Am Board Fam Med.* 2013;26(4):409–420.

86. Hollinger-Samson N, Pearson JL. The relationship between staff empathy and depressive symptoms in nursing home residents. *Aging Ment Health.* 2000;4:56–65.

87. Fogarty LA, Curbow BA, Wingard JR, McDonnell K, Somerfield MR. Can 40 seconds of compassion reduce patient anxiety? *J Clin Oncol.* 1999;17(1):371–379.

88. Neumann M, Wirtz M, Bollschweiler E, et al. Determinants and patient-reported long-term outcomes of physician empathy in oncology: A structural equation modelling approach. *Patient Educ Couns.* 2007;69(1–3):63–75.

89. Zachariae R, Pedersen CG, Jensen AB, Ehrnrooth E, Rossen PB, von der Maase H. Association of perceived physician communication style with patient satisfaction, distress, cancer-related self-efficacy, and perceived control over the disease. *Br J Cancer.* 2003;88(5):658–665.

90. Dibbelt S, Schaidhammer M, Fleischer C, Greitemann B. [Patient-doctor interaction in rehabilitation: Is there a relationship between perceived interaction quality and long term treatment results?]. *Rehabilitation (Stuttg).* 2010;49(5):315–325.

91. van Osch M, Sep M, van Vliet LM, van Dulmen S, Bensing JM. Reducing patients' anxiety and uncertainty, and improving recall in bad news consultations. *Health Psychol.* 2014;33(11):1382–1390.

92. Sep MS, van Osch M, van Vliet LM, Smets EM, Bensing JM. The power of clinicians' affective communication: How reassurance about non-abandonment can reduce patients' physiological arousal and increase information recall in bad news consultations. An experimental study using analogue patients. *Patient Educ Couns.* 2014;95(1):45–52.

93. Verheul W, Sanders A, Bensing J. The effects of physicians' affect-oriented communication style and raising expectations on analogue patients' anxiety, affect and expectancies. *Patient Educ Couns.* 2010;80(3):300–306.

94. Weiss R, Vittinghoff E, Fang MC, et al. Associations of physician empathy with patient anxiety and ratings of communication in hospital admission encounters. *J Hosp Med.* 2017;12(10):805–810.

95. Lelorain S, Bredart A, Dolbeault S, Sultan S. A systematic review of the associations between empathy measures and patient outcomes in cancer care. *Psychooncology.* 2012;21(12):1255–1264.

96. Roberts CS, Cox CE, Reintgen DS, Baile WF, Gibertini M. Influence of physician communication on newly diagnosed breast patients' psychologic adjustment and decision-making. *Cancer.* 1994;74(1 Suppl):336–341.

97. Mager WM, Andrykowski MA. Communication in the cancer "bad news" consultation: Patient perceptions and psychological adjustment. *Psychooncology.* 2002;11(1):35–46.

98. Shanafelt TD, Bowen DA, Venkat C, et al. The physician–patient relationship and quality of life: Lessons from chronic lymphocytic leukemia. *Leuk Res.* 2009;33(2):263–270.

99. Ong LM, Visser MR, Lammes FB, de Haes JC. Doctor–patient communication and cancer patients' quality of life and satisfaction. *Patient Educ Couns.* 2000;41(2):145–156.

100. Little P, White P, Kelly J, Everitt H, Mercer S. Randomised controlled trial of a brief intervention targeting predominantly non-verbal communication in general practice consultations. *Br J Gen Pract.* 2015;65(635):e351–356.

101. Roter DL, Hall JA, Kern DE, Barker LR, Cole KA, Roca RP. Improving physicians' interviewing skills and reducing patients' emotional distress: A randomized clinical trial. *Arch Intern Med.* 1995;155(17):1877–1884.

102. Mercer SW, Neumann M, Wirtz M, Fitzpatrick B, Vojt G. General practitioner empathy, patient enablement, and patient-reported outcomes in primary care in an area of high socio-economic deprivation in Scotland: A pilot prospective study using structural equation modeling. *Patient Educ Couns.* 2008;73(2):240–245.

103. Barefoot JC, Brummett BH, Williams RB, et al. Recovery expectations and long-term prognosis of patients with coronary heart disease. *Arch Intern Med.* 2011;171(10):929–935.

104. Mondloch MV, Cole DC, Frank JW. Does how you do depend on how you think you'll do? A systematic review of the evidence for a relation between patients' recovery expectations and health outcomes. *CMAJ.* 2001;165:174–179.

105. Zolnierek KB, Dimatteo MR. Physician communication and patient adherence to treatment: A meta-analysis. *Med Care.* 2009;47(8):826–834.

106. Hall JA, Roter DL, Katz NR. Meta-analysis of correlates of provider behavior in medical encounters. *Med Care.* 1988;26(7):657–675.

107. Beach MC, Keruly J, Moore RD. Is the quality of the patient–provider relationship associated with better adherence and health outcomes for patients with HIV? *J Gen Intern Med.* 2006;21(6):661–665.

108. Heszen-Klemens I, Lapinska E. Doctor–patient interaction, patients' health behavior and effects of treatment. *Soc Sci Med.* 1984;19(1): 9–18.
109. Mercer SW, Jani BD, Maxwell M, Wong SY, Watt GC. Patient enablement requires physician empathy: A cross-sectional study of general practice consultations in areas of high and low socioeconomic deprivation in Scotland. *BMC Fam Pract.* 2012;13:6.
110. Fuertes JN, Boylan LS, Fontanella JA. Behavioral indices in medical care outcome: The working alliance, adherence, and related factors. *J Gen Intern Med.* 2009;24(1):80–85.
111. Bennett JK, Fuertes JN, Keitel M, Phillips R. The role of patient attachment and working alliance on patient adherence, satisfaction, and health-related quality of life in lupus treatment. *Patient Educ Couns.* 2011;85(1):53–59.
112. Francis V, Korsch BM, Morris MJ. Gaps in doctor–patient communication. Patients' response to medical advice. *N Engl J Med.* 1969;280(10):535–540.
113. Kerse N, Buetow S, Mainous AG, 3rd, Young G, Coster G, Arroll B. Physician–patient relationship and medication compliance: A primary care investigation. *Ann Fam Med.* 2004;2(5):455–461.
114. Mahmoudian A, Zamani A, Tavakoli N, Farajzadegan Z, Fathollahi-Dehkordi F. Medication adherence in patients with hypertension: Does satisfaction with doctor-patient relationship work? *J Res Med Sci.* 2017;22:48.
115. Kahn KL, Schneider EC, Malin JL, Adams JL, Epstein AM. Patient centered experiences in breast cancer: Predicting long-term adherence to tamoxifen use. *Med Care.* 2007;45(5):431–439.
116. Wilkinson H, Whittington R, Perry L, Eames C. Examining the relationship between burnout and empathy in healthcare professionals: A systematic review. *Burn Res.* 2017;6:18–29.
117. Gleichgerrcht E, Decety J. Empathy in clinical practice: How individual dispositions, gender, and experience moderate empathic concern, burnout, and emotional distress in physicians. *PLoS One.* 2013;8(4):e61526.
118. Dasan S, Gohil P, Cornelius V, Taylor C. Prevalence, causes and consequences of compassion satisfaction and compassion fatigue in emergency care: A mixed-methods study of UK NHS Consultants. *Emerg Med J.* 2015;32(8):588–594.
119. Shanafelt TD, West C, Zhao X, et al. Relationship between increased personal well-being and enhanced empathy among internal medicine residents. *J Gen Intern Med.* 2005;20(7):559–564.
120. Thomas MR, Dyrbye LN, Huntington JL, et al. How do distress and well-being relate to medical student empathy? A multicenter study. *J Gen Intern Med.* 2007;22(2):177–183.

121. Lamothe M, Boujut E, Zenasni F, Sultan S. To be or not to be empathic: The combined role of empathic concern and perspective taking in understanding burnout in general practice. *BMC Fam Pract.* 2014;15:15.

122. Tei S, Becker C, Kawada R, et al. Can we predict burnout severity from empathy-related brain activity? *Transl Psychiatry.* 2014;4:e393.

123. Bourgault P, Lavoie S, Paul-Savoie E, et al. Relationship between empathy and well-being among emergency nurses. *J Emerg Nurs.* 2015;41(4):323–328.

124. Mascaro JS, Kelley S, A. D, et al. Meditation buffers medical student compassion from the deleterious effects of depression. *J Posit Psychol.* 2018;13:133–142.

125. Krasner MS, Epstein RM, Beckman H, et al. Association of an educational program in mindful communication with burnout, empathy, and attitudes among primary care physicians. *JAMA.* 2009;302(12):1284–1293.

126. McClelland LE, Gabriel AS, DePuccio MJ. Compassion practices, nurse well-being, and ambulatory patient experience ratings. *Med Care.* 2018;56(1):4–10.

127. Barsade SG, O'Neill OA. What's love got to do with it? A longitudinal study of the culture of companionate love and employee and client outcomes in a long-term care setting. *Adm Sci Q.* 2014;59:551–598.

128. Brazeau CM, Schroeder R, Rovi S, Boyd L. Relationships between medical student burnout, empathy, and professionalism climate. *Acad Med.* 2010;85(10 Suppl):S33–36.

129. Chen KY, Yang CM, Lien CH, et al. Burnout, job satisfaction, and medical malpractice among physicians. *Int J Med Sci.* 2013;10(11):1471–1478.

130. Weng HC, Hung CM, Liu YT, et al. Associations between emotional intelligence and doctor burnout, job satisfaction and patient satisfaction. *Med Educ.* 2011;45(8):835–842.

131. Derksen F, Bensing J, Kuiper S, van Meerendonk M, Lagro-Janssen A. Empathy: What does it mean for GPs? A qualitative study. *Fam Pract.* 2015;32(1):94–100.

132. Gleichgerrcht E, Decety J. The relationship between different facets of empathy, pain perception and compassion fatigue among physicians. *Front Behav Neurosci.* 2014;8:243.

133. Wiens K, McKee A. Why some people get burned out and others don't. *Harv Bus Rev.* 2016;94(11). https://hbr.org/2016/11/why-some-people-get-burned-out-and-others-dont

134. McKee A, Wiens K. Prevent burnout by making compassion a habit. *Harv Bus Rev.* 2017;95(3). https://hbr.org/2017/05/prevent-burnout-by-making-compassion-a-habit

135. West CP, Tan AD, Habermann TM, Sloan JA, Shanafelt TD. Association of resident fatigue and distress with perceived medical errors. *JAMA.* 2009;302(12):1294–1300.

136. West CP, Huschka MM, Novotny PJ, et al. Association of perceived medical errors with resident distress and empathy: A prospective longitudinal study. *JAMA*. 2006;296(9):1071–1078.

137. Shanafelt TD, Bradley KA, Wipf JE, Back AL. Burnout and self-reported patient care in an internal medicine residency program. *Ann Intern Med*. 2002;136(5):358–367.

138. Shanafelt TD, Balch CM, Bechamps G, et al. Burnout and medical errors among American surgeons. *Ann Surg*. 2010;251(6):995–1000.

139. Welp A, Meier LL, Manser T. The interplay between teamwork, clinicians' emotional exhaustion, and clinician-rated patient safety: A longitudinal study. *Crit Care*. 2016;20(1):110.

140. Sokol-Hessner L, Folcarelli PH, Sands KE. Emotional harm from disrespect: The neglected preventable harm. *BMJ Qual Saf*. 2015;24(9):550–553.

141. Casalino LP, Gans D, Weber R, et al. US physician practices spend more than $15.4 billion annually to report quality measures. *Health Aff (Millwood)*. 2016;35(3):401–406.

142. Masso Guijarro P, Aranaz Andres JM, Mira JJ, Perdiguero E, Aibar C. Adverse events in hospitals: The patient's point of view. *Qual Saf Health Care*. 2010;19(2):144–147.

143. Kuzel AJ, Woolf SH, Gilchrist VJ, et al. Patient reports of preventable problems and harms in primary health care. *Ann Fam Med*. 2004;2(4):333–340.

144. Kraft-Todd GT, Reinero DA, Kelley JM, Heberlein AS, Baer L, Riess H. Empathic nonverbal behavior increases ratings of both warmth and competence in a medical context. *PLoS One*. 2017;12(5):e0177758.

145. van Vliet LM, van der Wall E, Albada A, Spreeuwenberg PM, Verheul W, Bensing JM. The validity of using analogue patients in practitioner-patient communication research: Systematic review and meta-analysis. *J Gen Intern Med*. 2012;27(11):1528–1543.

146. Ogle J, Bushnell JA, Caputi P. Empathy is related to clinical competence in medical care. *Med Educ*. 2013;47(8):824–831.

147. Toi M, Batson CD. More evidence that empathy is a source of altruistic motivation. *J Pers Soc Psychol*. 1982;43:281–292.

148. Batson CD, Duncan BD, Ackerman P, Buckley T, Birch K. Is empathic emotion a source of altruistic motivation? *J Pers Soc Psychol*. 1981;40:290–302.

149. Slepian ML, Kirby JN. To whom do we confide our secrets? *Pers Soc Psychol Bull*. 2018;44(7):1008–1023.

150. McClelland LE, Vogus TJ. Compassion practices and HCAHPS: Does rewarding and supporting workplace compassion influence patient perceptions? *Health Serv Res*. 2014;49(5):1670–1683.

151. Betts D, Balan-Cohen A, Shukla M, Kumar N. *The Value of Patient Experience: Hospitals with Better Patient-Reported Experience Perform Better Financially*. Washington, DC: Deloitte Center for Health Solutions; 2016.

152. HealthTap. Survey reveals 85 percent of patients choose compassion over pricing when choosing a doctor. https://www.businesswire.com/news/home/20180206005704/en/Survey-Reveals-85-Percent-Patients-Choose-Compassion Published February 6, 2018.

153. Dignity Health. Americans rate kindness as top factor in care. https://www.dignityhealth.org/about-us/press-center/press-releases/majority-of-americans-rate-kindness Published November 13, 2013.

154. Menendez ME, Chen NC, Mudgal CS, Jupiter JB, Ring D. Physician empathy as a driver of hand surgery patient satisfaction. *J Hand Surg Am.* 2015;40(9):1860–1865 e1862.

155. Hojat M, Louis DZ, Maxwell K, Markham FW, Wender RC, Gonnella JS. A brief instrument to measure patients' overall satisfaction with primary care physicians. *Fam Med.* 2011;43(6):412–417.

156. Comstock LM, Hooper EM, Goodwin JM, Goodwin JS. Physician behaviors that correlate with patient satisfaction. *J Med Educ.* 1982;57(2):105–112.

157. Trzeciak S, Gaughan JP, Bosire J, Angelo M, Holzberg AS, Mazzarelli AJ. Association between Medicare star ratings for patient experience and Medicare spending per beneficiary for US hospitals. *J Patient Exp.* 2017;4(1):17–21.

158. Stewart M, Brown JB, Donner A, et al. The impact of patient-centered care on outcomes. *J Fam Pract.* 2000;49(9):796–804.

159. Bertakis KD, Azari R. Patient-centered care is associated with decreased health care utilization. *J Am Board Fam Med.* 2011;24(3):229–239.

160. Epstein RM, Franks P, Shields CG, et al. Patient-centered communication and diagnostic testing. *Ann Fam Med.* 2005;3(5):415–421.

161. Little P, Everitt H, Williamson I, et al. Observational study of effect of patient centredness and positive approach on outcomes of general practice consultations. *BMJ.* 2001;323(7318):908–911.

162. Shanafelt T, Goh J, Sinsky C. The business case for investing in physician well-being. *JAMA Intern Med.* 2017;177(12):1826–1832.

163. Bureau of Labor Statistics. *Number and Percent Distribution of Nonfatal Occupational Injuries and Illnesses Involving Days Away from Work by Nature of Injury or Illness and Number of Days Away from Work.* Washington, DC: BLS; 2001.

164. American Psychological Association. *Stress in America.* Washington, DC: APA; 2007.

165. American Psychological Association. *Psychologically Healthy Workplace Program Fact Sheet: By the Numbers.* Washington, DC: APA, 2008.

166. Beckman HB, Markakis KM, Suchman AL, Frankel RM. The doctor-patient relationship and malpractice. Lessons from plaintiff depositions. *Arch Intern Med.* 1994;154(12):1365–1370.

167. Hickson GB, Clayton EW, Entman SS, et al. Obstetricians' prior malpractice experience and patients' satisfaction with care. *JAMA.* 1994;272(20):1583–1587.

168. Slawson PF. Psychiatric malpractice: Some aspects of cause. *Psychiatr Hosp.* 1984;15(3):141–144.
169. Vincent C, Young M, Phillips A. Why do people sue doctors? A study of patients and relatives taking legal action. *Lancet.* 1994;343(8913):1609–1613.
170. Moore PJ, Adler NE, Robertson PA. Medical malpractice: The effect of doctor-patient relations on medical patient perceptions and malpractice intentions. *West J Med.* 2000;173(4):244–250.

8

A Wholistic Approach to a Compassionate and Flourishing Life

As a physician-educator who has worked in healthcare for more than 30 years, I have served numerous patients and worked with many healthcare professionals, caregivers, and physicians-in-training. As a chaplain, I have talked to many inmates, palliative care patients, and other chaplains. As I serve in these capacities, I have witnessed the many joys and sufferings of our human existence. I have also been humbled to see the strength, courage, and resilience that humans demonstrate despite the trials and tribulations of life. I have pondered deeply on what it takes to transform the obstacles to compassion into opportunities for our growth and development, as well as the additional ingredients that are essential for leading a compassionate, flourishing life.

Psychological Well-Being

As we become more aware, more attuned, and more reflective, we may discover many uncharted territories that pose difficulties. Counselling (or coaching, psychotherapy) can bring about additional clarity, openness, and deep healing. By talking to a trained professional, we can express thoughts and feelings that could not be shared with our loved ones or friends. Talking to a professional also allows our two hemispheres to process and integrate difficult experiences, thoughts, and emotions. Neuroscience has shown that the right side of our brain processes emotions and autobiographical memories and often causes us stress through ruminating mental activities. By putting our experience into words and the details of a memory in order, the left side of the brain helps us to make sense of our feelings and recollections. In this way, we can respond to setbacks in a healthy way.[1] Talking to a professional is also a co-creative process. It offers us new perspectives on our habitual thinking style, so that we can find a novel creative approach to handle life situations and relationships through a combination of reframing, decentring, and repatterning.

For some of us who may have been exposed to sufferings at a very young age, psychological wounds could leave a strong imprint in our physical, mental, emotional, and psychosocial being. In this situation, mindfulness practices, compassion training, and cultivation of inner compassion may not be sufficient to unblock our deep, unconscious psychological defenses against raw, painful wounds. In this regard, psychotherapy can help point out and unravel the defenses that we have erected so that they gradually lose their hold on us. It also guards us against "spiritual bypass"; that is, using spiritual ideas and practices to evade or avoid facing unresolved emotional issues, psychological trauma, and unfinished developmental tasks.[2]

Psychotherapy also helps us develop authentic self-expression as mature adults. Therapy that incorporates the need for "secure attachment"—safety, compassion, nonjudgment, and mirroring—and that nurtures authenticity can help us rediscover our basic goodness. It helps us identify our unique talents and develop a genuine expression of our innate capacities as self-actualized mature adults so that we can transcend self-focused needs and increase compassionate actions.

Ethics and Moral Resilience

As healthcare professionals, we are often confronted with conflicting moral demands, uncertainties about the proper course of action, and real or perceived inability to do the "right" thing in the face of time pressure, limited resources, and power hierarchy. Cultivating moral resilience is key to upholding our values and maintaining our integrity.[3] Moral resilience is "the capacity of individuals to sustain or restore their integrity in response to moral complexity, confusion, distress, or setbacks."[4] It is "the ability and willingness to speak, to take right and good action, in the face of an adversity that is moral/ethical in nature."[5]

What does it take to cultivate moral resilience? Recognizing moral challenges and moral development are essential.

Making ethical decisions requires us first to recognize moral challenges, which may take three forms: moral uncertainty, conflict, and dilemma.[6-9] *Moral uncertainty* occurs when one is unable to define the moral issue at stake or is unsure about which moral principles to apply.[6,7] *Moral conflict* arises when there is tension between two or more moral values or principles, when disagreement exists about which moral values or principles apply, or when there is confusion about the appropriate course of action.[9,10] *Moral dilemma* happens when two or more moral principles clearly apply, but they support conflicting courses of action.[9,10] These actions often can lead to tragic choices, serious harms, or moral crisis.

James Rest, an American psychologist, advanced a four-component model of moral development to deal with moral challenges. The four components are moral sensitivity, moral judgment/reasoning, moral motivation, and moral character/courage.[11] *Moral sensitivity* is the ability to recognize, frame, and contextualize an ethical situation. It involves the capacity to determine the form of moral challenges that one is facing and to identify morally pertinent features in a situation. *Moral judgment/reasoning* involves analyzing ethical issues, identifying choices, considering stakeholder interests, balancing consequences, weighing competing values and responsibilities, determining courses of action, and developing a rigorous rationale for action. *Moral motivation* (and identity formation) entails prioritizing ethical values and committing to take ethical action. It also leads to the development of professional identity that is aligned with professional values and codes of conduct. Last, *moral courage/character* entails executing ethical action, having the courage to follow one's convictions, persevering despite obstacles, and demonstrating audacity in the face of resistance.[11,12]

As healthcare professionals, we need to be aware of *moral remainder*—even when an ethically sound choice is prioritized, selected, and acted upon, there often are other imperative ethical values and principles that are left unmet.[8] This awareness is important to prevent us from falling into disappointment, moral distress, or burnout, and it enables us to accept, hold, and make peace with life's inevitable paradoxes. In addition to cultivating moral resilience at an individual level, we also need to create a culture for moral resilience and ethical practice at the organizational and system levels using a sustained and multifaceted approach.[13]

What does moral resilience look like to me, and how do I sustain it? Following the precepts has been instrumental for me to maintain my integrity, to be in touch with my deepest values, and to connect to who I am. There are different types of precepts that one may follow. For example, I often adhere to the Golden Rule—"Do unto others as you would have them do unto you"—as my "North Star precept," a term I heard from Sensei Hozan Alan Senauke, to navigate the water of life. Religious vows, such as the Ten Commandments common to the Abrahamic religions and the Five Buddhist Precepts,[14] are also useful for those who follow a particular spiritual tradition. Interestingly, the Five Buddhist Precepts (i.e., abstain from killing, stealing, sexual misconduct, lying, and intoxication) overlap with those found in the Ten Commandments. Indeed, philosophers of ethics regard these five precepts as universal because the first four, and sometimes the fifth, appear in many moral codes around the world throughout the ages.

These five precepts may seem to be quite straightforward to follow. However, after practising and integrating them into my life for a while, I have come to realize that they are not as easy to keep as I once thought. Indeed, as I use them to observe, investigate, and guide my everyday actions in my body, speech, and mind, layer upon layer of their subtle meanings begin to unveil. For example, I come to see that the precept of not killing does not only affirm the preciousness of life, it also points us more broadly to do no harm, no matter how justifiable it may seem on the surface. When I encounter a difficult person or situation, I ask myself: Am I holding resentment, rage, or revenge with an intention to harm? In a moment of anger, self-righteousness, or defensiveness, have I ever harboured a murderous impulse—even just for a brief moment—to those I consider to be slighting, disrespecting, or insulting me? How can I transform the energy of anger, using it as a teacher to guide me into non-reactivity and non-harming, so that I can act most skilfully? At a deeper level, this precept asks us to reflect on the interconnectedness and interdependence of all things and calls upon us to live in harmony with everything, whether humans, animals, plants, animate or inanimate objects, or our planet.

How about the precept of not stealing? While it asks us to refrain from taking anything not given, it also urges us to examine whether we foster a mind of poverty. I ask myself: Have I turned a blind eye on someone in need—a homeless person, a beggar on the street, a colleague in distress—because I feel that I am not able to help, that it is too painful to meet their eyes, or that I do not have the strength to even acknowledge their struggle and personhood? How can I use all the ingredients of my life, giving my best effort, while at the same time be willing to ask and accept what is needed? At a deeper level, when we truly experience the oneness of all things, there is really no giver nor receiver: the act of giving and receiving is simply the universe rearranging itself.

Similarly, the precept of refraining from sexual misconduct asks us to treat all beings with respect and dignity. I ask: How can I maintain an authentic and intimate presence with someone I am fond of, without using or clinging? How can I perceive that there is really no separation between myself and others and that there is no need for me to fill this illusory gap out of my fear, insecurity, and ignorance? Roshi Reb Anderson pointed out, at a deeper level, that this precept doesn't say sexuality is bad or good. Rather, it reveals that by "neither identifying with nor distancing ourselves from our sexuality, we gradually become intimate with it. From this intimacy, appropriate sexual conduct spontaneously emerges."[15]

The precept of non-lying not only asks us to be truthful; it also directs us to be transparent. I ask: How can I be transparent to my inner life, including my conditioning, biases, and fear? How can I make the world transparent to me by seeing things with clarity from a deep inner stillness? How can I be transparent to the world no matter how vulnerable it may make me feel? Roshi Joan Halifax called this the "threefold transparency": being self-transparent, making the world transparent to us, and being transparent to the world.[16] At a deeper level, the precept of speaking truthfully asks us to acknowledge with humility that there is really no one truth in the ordinary realm as our views are necessarily incomplete based on our limited perception. This is captured aptly by the axiom: "Where there is perception, there is deception."[17]

Last, the precept of not being intoxicated asks us to look at what "nutriments"—healthy or unhealthy—we allow into our body and mind. I ask myself: Why do I choose not to use cigarettes, alcohol, or illicit drugs? Knowing that the messages from some world leaders are toxic, why do I still watch or listen to the news regularly, almost to the point of addiction and obsession? Are my actions motivated by the pursuits of wealth, fame, or possessions? Does my mind harbour negative, greedy, or aversive thoughts from time to time? Thich Nhat Hahn called these the "four nutriments"—edible food (including alcohol and illicit drugs), sense impression (the six senses), action (volition), and consciousness (thoughts)—and alerted us to how they can lead to happiness or suffering. At a deeper level, we may find that the reason we allow unhealthy nutriments to enter our system is that we are dissatisfied with our current experience and are trying to mask it, suppress it, or run away from it. Ultimately, this precept is about letting go of all our self-concerns and appreciating all things as they are.[15]

Social Engagement

A truly transformative approach to living a compassionate life and to reaching our full human potential needs to address not only our personal relations to suffering, but also acknowledge that personal suffering has societal causes. As an inner practice, mindfulness and compassion/loving-kindness provide clarity, courage, and a stable grounding so that one can turn outward to support or engage in actions that address different issues in one's own environment or in the larger world. These issues could include interpersonal relations, workplace conflicts, social injustice, inequity, racism, discrimination, poverty, and environmental devastation.

When we look deeply, as individuals and a society as a whole, we have often failed to acknowledge or bear witness to the fact that racism, poverty, violence, and injustice are alive, real, and dangerous. Many of us may have conditioned ourselves to deny the existence of or avoided dealing with these issues, perhaps because when we experience them, fear overwhelms us—fear of our own prejudice and guilt, fear of our incompetence to address them, and fear of calling out the perpetrators.

However, through our silence, our inaction, and our choosing to live with blinders on in a comfortable, conditioned state of ignorance, we have unwittingly perpetuated untold cycles of injustices and sufferings. It is important to keep in mind that, ultimately, we can only experience a true sense of wholeness—both personally and collectively—in an inclusive, just, and harmonious society in which everyone flourishes.

To confront these social issues, courage, moral nerve, and strength are necessary. The word "courage" derives from the Latin word *cor* or heart, and from *corage* in Old French. Courage does not mean that we do not have fear, but rather that we follow our hearts to do the right thing in spite of fear. As Nelson Mandela said: "Courage was not the absence of fear, but the triumph over it."[18] By listening deeply to our hearts, principled compassionate action will spontaneously emerge. According to Roshi Joan Halifax, principled compassionate action "is a rigorous, balanced stance of a 'strong back' of equanimity that allows one to be clear, courageous, and principled amid the most challenging circumstances with the 'soft front' of open-heartedness, kindness, and empathy leading to compassion."[19] Its hallmark includes "leveraging one's moral outrage by executing unpopular decisions and when appropriate, conscientiously objecting to ethically compromising situations, despite resistance, in a fair, modulated manner."[19] Whether it is in service to social justice, nonviolence, or peace, principled compassionate action reminds us what we stand for supports us to stay true to our deepest values and prompts us to act in accordance to who we really are.

What does principled compassionate action look like to me? I recall a recent event in which one of the academic leaders in my institution, out of "good-hearted humour," made a series of misogynist and racist comments. It created an uproar immediately, especially among the residents and early to mid-career women faculty. They wanted to speak up but were hesitant because of the power hierarchy and fear of being reprimanded. I asked them: What is your intention? Is it primarily to make your upset or frustration known? Is it to punish, retaliate, or humiliate the speaker? What principles are at stake here? Could we turn this ordeal into a learning opportunity, not just for the speaker, but also for everyone involved? I reminded them that it is not time to act when there is any indignation, self-righteousness, and victimization within us. I also pointed out that privilege is often invisible to people in the dominant group who have it and that our job is to learn and practise the skills of challenging oppressive remarks, behaviours, policies, and institutional structures without causing harm or falling into self-righteousness. From a place of calmness, they shared their concerns earnestly with the top leaders. I was pleasantly surprised that the speaker was completely appalled by his remarks and took immediate action to apologize to the entire department with candor, courage, and grace. In fact, it was the first time, in my 25 years in the department, that I witnessed a complaint of this nature being handled so swiftly, seriously, and genuinely by our leaders. I learned from this ordeal that each of us can take steps to help create a more just, inclusive, and compassionate workplace, culture, and society wherever we are.

A Transcendental Life

Finally, as the famous American psychologist Abraham Maslow noted,[20,21] an integrated, fulfilling approach to living predicates upon meeting eight hierarchical levels of human needs: (1) physiological—food, water, warmth, rest; (2) safety and security; (3) love and belonging—friendship, intimacy, family, sense of connection; (4) esteem—respect, recognition, sense of accomplishment; (5) cognitive—knowledge and understanding, curiosity, exploration; (6) aesthetic—appreciation and search for beauty, balance, form; (7) self-actualization—realizing personal potential, self-fulfillment, seeking personal growth and peak experiences; and (8) transcendence—experiences with nature and aesthetics, mystical experiences, service to others, meaning and purpose, wisdom. In this regard, psychological well-being, moral resilience, and social engagement build the foundation and act synergistically so that we can gradually move beyond self-centredness and our existential sufferings. From there, mindful awareness, loving-kindness, and compassion allow us to respond to life circumstances from a still, inner space that is deeper than our personality and our conceptual mind, a place from which we draw strength and wisdom. And as our practice and insights deepen, we can begin to realize the true nature of reality; appreciate the suchness of all phenomena that transcend all notions, concepts, and ideas; and experience a sense of wholeness, deep joy, and peace.

Summary of Key Points

- Counselling, coaching, and psychotherapy can bring about additional clarity, openness, and deep healing. They help us to develop a genuine expression of our innate capacities as self-actualized mature adults, so that we can transcend self-focused needs and increase compassionate actions.
- Moral resilience is one's capacity to maintain or restore integrity in face of moral complexity, confusion, distress, or failures. It requires one to have the ability to recognize moral challenges and train in moral development. One effective way to build moral resilience is to follow the precepts.
- Moral challenges include moral uncertainty, conflict, and dilemma. *Moral uncertainty* occurs when one is unable to define the moral issue at stake or is unsure about which moral principles to apply. *Moral conflict* arises when there is tension between two or more moral values or principles, when disagreement exists about which moral values or principles apply, or when there is confusion about the appropriate course of action. *Moral dilemma* happens when two or more moral principles clearly apply, but they support conflicting courses of action.
- Moral development consists of four components: moral sensitivity, judgment/reasoning, motivation, and character/courage. *Moral sensitivity* is the ability to recognize, frame, and contextualize an ethical situation. *Moral judgment/reasoning* involves analyzing ethical issues, considering stakeholder interests, balancing consequences, weighing competing values and responsibilities, determining courses of action, and developing a rigorous rationale for action. *Moral motivation* entails prioritizing ethical values and committing to take ethical action. *Moral courage/character* involves executing ethical action, having the courage to follow one's convictions, persevering despite obstacles, and demonstrating audacity in the face of resistance.

- It is important for healthcare professionals to be aware of and regulate *moral remainder*; that is, even when an ethically sound choice is prioritized, selected, and acted upon, there often are other imperative ethical values and principles that are left unmet.
- A truly transformative approach to living a compassionate life and to reaching our full human potential needs to address not only our personal relations to suffering, but also acknowledge that personal suffering has societal causes. Ultimately, we can only experience a true sense of wholeness—both personally and collectively—in an inclusive, just, and harmonious society in which everyone flourishes.
- Principled compassionate action is "a rigorous, balanced stance of a 'strong back' of equanimity that allows one to be clear, courageous, and principled amid the most challenging circumstances with the 'soft front' of open-heartedness, kindness, and empathy leading to compassion." It leverages "one's moral outrage by executing unpopular decisions and when appropriate, conscientiously objecting to ethically compromising situations, despite resistance, in a fair, modulated manner."

References

1. Siegel DJ, Bryson TP. *The Whole-Brain Child: 12 Revolutionary Strategies to Nurture Your Child's Developing Mind.* New York: Delacorte Press; 2011.
2. Flics D. What meditation can't cure. In: Melvin McLeod, Tynette Deveaux, ed. *Buddhadharma: The Practitioner's Quarterly.* Boulder, CO: Shambhala Publications; 2017:65–71.
3. Rushton CH, Kaszniak AW, Halifax J. Cultivating Essential Capacities for Moral Resilience. In: Rushton CH, ed. *Moral Resilience: Transforming Moral Suffering in Healthcare.* New York: Oxford University Press; 2018:150–182.
4. Rushton CH. Moral resilience: A capacity for navigating moral distress in critical care. *AACN Adv Crit Care.* 2016;27(1):111–119.
5. Lachman VD. Moral resilience: Managing and preventing moral distress and moral residue. *Medsurg Nurs.* 2016;25(2):121–124.
6. Lockhart L. *Moral Uncertainty and Its Consequences.* New York: Oxford University Press; 2000.
7. Krister B. Moral uncertainty. *Philosophy Compass.* 2017 12(3):e12408.

8. Jameton A. *Nursing Practice: The Ethical Issues.* Englewood Cliffs, NJ: Prentice-Hall; 1984.

9. McConnell T. Moral dilemmas. Stanford Encyclopedia of Philosophy. https://plato.stanford.edu/entries/moral-dilemmas/#ConMorDil Published 2018.

10. Jameton A. Dilemmas of moral distress: Moral responsibility and nursing practice. *AWHONNS Clin Issues Perinat Womens Health Nurs.* 1993;4:542–555.

11. Rest J. The Major Components of Morality. In: Kurtines W, Gewortz J, eds. *Morality, Moral Development, and Moral Behavior.* New York: Wiley; 1984:24–38.

12. Rest JR, Narvaez D, Bebeau MJ, Thoma SJ. *Postconventional Moral Thinking: A Neo-Kohlbergian Approach.* Mahweh, NJ: Lawrence Erlbaum Associates; 1999.

13. Rushton CH, Sharma M. Creating a Culture of Moral Resilience and Ethical Practice. In: Rushton CH, ed. *Moral Resilience: Transforming Moral Suffering in Healthcare.* New York: Oxford University Press; 2018:243–280.

14. Upaya. The sixteen practices of a Zen peacemaker. https://www.upaya.org/teachings/liturgy/peacemaking/

15. Anderson R. *Being Upright: Zen Meditation and Bodhisattva Precepts.* Boulder, CO: Shambhala; 2001.

16. Halifax J. *Being with Dying: Cultivating Compassion and Fearlessness in the Presence of Death.* Boston, MA: Shambhala; 2009.

17. Thich Nhat Hahn. *The Heart of the Buddha's Teaching: Transforming Suffering into Peace, Joy, and Liberation.* New York: Harmony Books; 2015.

18. Brainy Quote. Nelson mandela quotes brainyquote.com. BrainyMedia Inc; 2020. https://www.brainyquote.com/quotes/nelson_mandela_178789

19. Rushton CH, Kaszniak AW, Halifax JS. A framework for understanding moral distress among palliative care clinicians. *J Palliat Med.* 2013;16(9):1074–1079.

20. Maslow AH, Frager R. *Motivation and Personality.* 3rd ed. New York: Harper and Row; 1987.

21. Maslow AH. *Religions, Values and Peak-Experiences.* New York: Penguin; 1994.

Postface

In these pages, I have laid out the evolutional, biological, psychological, and spiritual basis of compassion, showing that it is deeply ingrained in our human nature. I have also shown that compassion is trainable and that the brain changes as we become kinder and more compassionate toward ourselves and others. I have described the obstacles to compassion and what it takes to cultivate a compassionate and flourishing life. You may ask: How do I start? What does compassion look like to you as you follow a different career trajectory to become a physician-chaplain? Although everyone's path is different, I would like to offer you some personal experiences from my journey.

Rites of Passage

In the Preface, I described the ordeal of my hearing loss 4 years ago, which I originally thought was the primary cause of the change in my career path. In retrospect, it was merely a catalyst as I was already going through a gradual shift in my life. About 8 years ago, I came across the book *Mindfulness: An Eight-Week Plan for Finding Peace in a Frantic World* by Professor Mark Williams (a co-founder of Mindfulness-Based Cognitive Therapy) and Danny Penman.[1] I followed the book's instruction and started to meditate for 8 minutes twice a day at the beginning and slowly increased to about 30 minutes daily. Over 8 weeks, I began to notice that I became less reactive, less judgmental, and more opened to new perspectives. Although I took up meditation originally to help with personal stress, I was surprised to find that I was quietly growing stronger and that I was changing as a doctor as well. I was more open to hear my patients' problems, more resourceful to serve them, and more consistent to act with kindness. After I finished the program, seeing the benefits of the practice, I made a commitment to meditate every day for the rest of my life.

At around the same time, I began to work with a communication consultant. I learned about the importance of making and keeping promises, taking responsibility, and using effective communication, as well as having a clear purpose in life. This work, together with my meditation practice, has allowed me to investigate many unexamined assumptions, my habitual thought patterns, and some psychological issues that I was unaware of.

With the unexpected hearing loss, I suddenly realized that although my work with the consultant has helped me to become a better, more effective, and empathic leader, it emphasized primarily the development of masculine qualities of "doing"—focused, goal-oriented, structured, logical, and driven. I began to realize that I need to *listen* to my body more because years of medical training have conditioned me to ignore my most basic bodily needs, let alone my overall physical health or my ability to attune to the deep inner messages and wisdom that my body carries. Therefore, I decided to work with a counsellor instead, in order to bring the masculine and feminine into greater balance by developing the feminine qualities of "being"—intuitive, receptive, fluid, allowing, and nurturing. I also began to explore my spiritual being in earnest, searching for the meaning and purpose of life, the experience of interconnectedness, and the values that are most important to me. In addition, I worked on some deep psychological wounds with my counsellor, a co-creative process that has allowed me to develop an authentic way of being despite the "noise" of the conventional world.

Then, about 3 years ago, I met Roshi Joan Halifax when she visited Toronto. I still remember vividly that, during our short conversation, one of the first things she told me was not to leave medicine, as I was seriously considering quitting at that time. After I completed the G.R.A.C.E. training with her, I decided to enter chaplaincy primarily as a path to grow spiritually and to prepare for other work outside of medicine. Little did I know that the training would completely open my eyes to the profound meaning of compassion, the importance of moral development, and the significance of social engagement. In addition to these insights, I discovered the importance of inner compassion. As Thich Nhat Hahn explained, mindfulness recognizes, embraces, and relieves our deep wounds.[2] By recognizing my own suffering with courage, I began to befriend my wounded inner child who has been "banished in the basement," hidden beneath my deep consciousness. By embracing her with tenderness, I invited the inner child to come up to the living room in my mindful presence and caring. By relieving difficult emotions, healing commenced. I began to discover how the deep roots of ignorance, attachment, and prejudice inside me have contributed not only to my own suffering but also to that of others. Through inner compassion, I came to realize our common humanity: just as I am, other beings are also suffering, they are also struggling with the same delusion, desire, and anger that I am wrestling with. And just as I am, other beings also want to be happy, they also want to lead a meaningful and purposeful life. From a place of deep sorrow and our shared humanity, I began to see that chaplaincy is an expression of my deep aspiration: to hear the cries of the world, to alleviate the pain and suffering of all by responding spontaneously, unconditionally, and appropriately.

Another significant insight I have gained is that living a contemplative life doesn't mean I need to be a recluse. With engaged mindfulness, I can actively engage in work that I am passionate about without losing myself in ego-gratification. Learning about systems thinking during chaplaincy training made me realize that I am part of the healthcare system—even if I turn away from it, I am still influencing it somehow. Despite its many challenges, I can be the first leverage point, tapping into the many years of professional training and the wealth of experience I have accumulated. I can look at the healthcare system as a fertile ground waiting for me to remove the weeds one at a time, water it with skilful means, and transform it into a beautiful garden. Although the garden may take a long time to bear fruit, I trust that my action will encourage others to address the many problems that healthcare professionals face and tackle the many issues that plague the system. At the same time, I realize that I am merely an instrument. I can endeavour to do my best while accepting that the outcomes may or may not be what I envision them to be.

From a larger perspective, I came to recognize that what I have gone through fits into a pattern of what the French ethnographer Arnold Van Gennep called "the rites of passage," characterized by three phases: separation, margin, and incorporation.[3] The separation phase usually begins when something comes to an end, whether it be a positive change or something that is difficult. In my case, the hearing loss triggered me to abandon my achieving, acquiring, and accumulating mode of living. During this phase, we may experience a sense of loss and grief as separation denotes that we are separating from something—either something unknown to ourselves or something that defines who we are. The second phase, the margin (liminality/ threshold/transition) phase, is a place of in-betweenness, of neither here nor there, of no longer belonging to the old but not yet of the new. It is characterized by ambiguity, uncertainty, anxiety, and hope. We may have question about ourselves, our relationships, our place in the world, and our purpose. Others may consider us "dangerous" or "polluting" as we do not fit into any traditional classifications and are regarded uncomfortably by the larger society.[4] Lying at the margins, we may feel quite vulnerable; however, this phase is both informative and potentially transformative. In my case, chaplaincy training has been a metamorphic experience to let go of my old "self," allowing my creativity, vitality, and beingness to come through with a new sense of clarity, possibility, and renewal. Now, as a physician-chaplain, I begin to enter the last phase, the incorporation phase, in which I consolidate what I have learned and implement new changes and insights into my life. I am also aware that this process of integration is often met with challenges as others may continue to see or expect me to be who I was, or they refuse to accept who I have become, or I may succumb to the seduction of past comfort. Writing this book on compassion has allowed me not only to share my experience, but also fulfill my intention in this new phase to focus on what truly matters in life.

The Three Tenets

What does compassion look like in my life? For me, a daily meditation practice is the principal support of my work in the world. Whether I am in the clinic, operating room, hospice, prison, or at home, the most important qualities that I endeavour to cultivate through meditative practice are a non-anxious presence, clarity of mind, and gentleness of heart. Instead of relying on prescribed techniques or a "compassionate persona" that masks my fear, uneasiness, or vulnerability, I remind myself to return again and again to the immediacy of whatever is happening, arising, and unfolding at this very moment. In this regard, the Three Tenets of the Zen Peacemakers (developed by the late Roshi Bernie Glassman and his wife Jishu Angyo Holmes)[5] have shown me the way to return to this immediacy again and again in many situations.

I learned about the Three Tenets of not knowing, bearing witness, and compassionate action from Roshi Joan Halifax.[6] The first tenet, *not knowing*, is the ability to be present in any situation without a preconceived agenda. It is a practice of letting go of fixed ideas about ourselves, others, and the universe. As I walk into the examining room, for example, I try to bring with me an "empty mind" or a "beginner's mind." This does not mean a "blank mind"; rather, I bring with me all that I have learned, all that I have experienced, and all that I am. Although I might have a plan in mind, I make sure that I listen carefully to what my patients have to say, bringing a sense of curiosity and openness to the encounter, and I pay close attention to the situation as it presents itself moment by moment before I decide on the next steps.

The second tenet, *bearing witness*, is the ability to see clearly the situation no matter how painful it is. I learned from Roshi Joan that the principle of "strong back" of equanimity and "soft front" of compassion[6] during formal meditative practice can also be applied in any daily situation. In healthcare, I have seen many colleagues adopting a matter-of-fact, professional demeanour, perhaps fearing that if they let themselves experience their patients' suffering, their hearts would break and they would not be able to carry out their work. Yet, as Mikel Monnett, a hospital chaplain, wrote: "In reality, if they would only allow their hearts to break—to fully experience the misery and suffering of their patients with them—they would find that an astonishing thing happens: their hearts can break and they can go on."[7] Bearing witness also means that we accept the joys and sufferings of this world as they are, without any preference, judgment, or attachment to outcomes.

Finally, for the third tenet, *compassionate* or *healing action*, I ask: "How can I truly serve?" I remind myself that patients are not equivalent to a *disease*—a "malfunctioning or maladaptation of biologic and psychophysiologic processes"—to be diagnosed and treated. Rather, they suffer from an *illness*—a human experience of sickness that "represents personal, interpersonal, and cultural reactions to disease or discomfort."[8] In addition to treating the disease, it is very important for me to help the patients and their families to work through their illness, recognizing that sometimes we may or may not be able to *cure*, yet, with loving-kindness and compassion, *healing* is always possible.

Being with Living and Dying

Cultivating a compassionate life is a life-long journey, with its ups and downs, dilemmas, and complexities, as well as its richness and challenges. I would like to share with you a personal story about an unexpected death of a close colleague and my experience supporting his wife during this very difficult time. I have changed their names here to protect their privacy.

Mark was a beloved mentor, a trusted colleague, and a wonderful friend who was always ready to listen, help, and offer witty, encouraging, and insightful words. I also became a friend of his wife, Anne, over many memorable conversations. About 5 years ago, both Mark and Anne were devastated by the death of their adult son in a tragic accident. Since then, I could feel a deep sense of unexpressed sorrow in them. I made sure to see them regularly to show them my concern, love, and support.

One morning about 3 years ago, I received the news that Mark had suffered from a massive stroke and was comatose in an intensive care unit while attending an out-of-province conference in Montreal. Knowing that Anne was alone in an unfamiliar city, I decided to fly to Montreal immediately despite my existing commitments. During the last 10 days of Mark's life, I had the opportunity to spend some very personal and intimate time with Anne. We went through ups and downs of our emotions, hopes and despair, moments of light-heartedness when we shared our stories, and we shed more than a few tears when we felt lost. We made many difficult decisions as best we could, hoping that they were the right ones—that Mark would have made the same decisions if he were able to tell us. And, ultimately, we had to let go; we accepted the inevitable and said our last goodbyes. I could still sense vividly the stillness after he took his last breath, Suffusing the room with an unfathomable peace and deep tranquility.

During these 10 intensely emotional days, I was keenly aware that I played several important roles: as a doctor, I helped Anne navigate the healthcare system and explained unfamiliar medical terminology and concepts to her; as a friend, I was someone whom Anne could lean on as she went through this stressful time, and I also served as a sounding board as she and their daughter made many difficult decisions; as a woman, I could identify with her the painful ordeal of first losing a treasured son and then her much-loved husband; and, as a colleague, I became the central messenger relaying Mark's latest development to colleagues in my department back home. All the while, I was also acutely aware that I had to balance these various demands on me carefully, as well as taking good care of myself in order to best serve my friends.

I remember that each day was a big unknown, with so many questions that swirled through my mind. Not knowing what would happen each day, each hour, each minute, how could I remain calm to provide the support that Anne needed without being cold or overly rational? Not knowing what the situation called for, how could I best serve Mark and Anne without pretending that I knew what was best for them individually and collectively? Not knowing whether a slightest movement of his toe was simply the release of a primitive reflexive movement which indicated a dire prognosis, or whether it was instead an indication that he was trying to communicate with us, how could I acknowledge Anne's observation without dashing her hopes but, at the same time, not losing touch with reality?

Bearing witness to Anne's loss and grief, how could I not be overwhelmed also by my own sadness while remaining strong and compassionate? Bearing witness to Anne's occasional bursts of anger over the course of Mark's demise—from the possibility of medication error that resulted in Mark's hemorrhagic stroke; to the intensivist's sudden decision to allow Mark to be transported back home to Toronto despite his coma, which brought Anne great joy only to have it reversed just as abruptly the following day; to the suggestion of withdrawing life support, which Anne equated with euthanasia—how could I acknowledge her frustrations without adding fuel to them, and how could I maintain my composure, gently guide her through reasoning without getting into a disagreement with her or disregarding her vulnerable state?

What were the most compassionate actions I could take during this difficult time? How could I respect Anne's privacy, dignity, and space, while ensuring that I was available when she needed me? How could I remain fully present, let go of any judgment or any preconceptions of what should or should not happen, and embrace each moment as it unfolded? How could I maintain a strong back, soft front as I cared for my friends?

While taking a break from the hospital one afternoon, as Anne and I strolled in a nearby park—watching a duck and its ducklings swimming in a pond, seeing a flock of birds hovering above us before soaring to the sky, hearing the trees whispering in the wind—I had a sudden, deeply felt appreciation that everything was constantly changing, that we were all intricately connected, and that we were surrounded by love and kindness.

During this ordeal, I was grateful that the Three Tenets, the teaching of "strong back, soft front," and a non-anxious presence became a guiding light for me each time I felt lost. I was also grateful that I could rely on my daily meditative practice which provided me with a solid foundation, a profound sense of grounding, and an unfathomable source of strength. I also learned that cultivating compassion is critical. I initially thought that turning part-time—seeing fewer patients so that I can spend more time on replenishing activities—was key for restoring my well-being. I now realize that it is the cultivation of compassion for others and myself, together with the practice of meditation and the search of wisdom, that have brought wholeness, deep joy, and peace to my life. Interestingly, two recent meta-analyses showed that "escapism" strategies (e.g., going part-time, taking vacation) have only modest effects on reducing burnout.[9,10]

A Koan

A *koan* is a succinct, paradoxical story, dialogue, question, or statement used in the Zen tradition as a meditation discipline to exhaust the analytical intellect, allowing the mind to come up with an appropriate response intuitively. I would like to share with you the following koan that invites us to experience for ourselves what compassion feels like. I encourage you to read it a few times, take a pause to see what arises, and perhaps jot down a few notes before continuing to read my thoughts and other commentaries on it.

Lingzhao's Helping (from 8th-century China)
One day, Layman Pang and his daughter, Lingzhao, were out selling bamboo baskets. Coming down off a bridge, the Layman stumbled and fell. When Lingzhao saw this, she ran to her father's side and threw herself to the ground. "What are you doing?" cried the Layman. "I saw you fall so I'm helping," replied Lingzhao. "Luckily no one was looking," remarked the Layman.

After reading this koan, you may ask: Why did Lingzhao run to her father's side and throw herself to the ground? How does that help? To me, Lingzhao's action signifies that she was willing to come alongside her father by meeting him where he was, to "lower" herself to see things from his perspective, and to not presume that she knew what would be the best course of actions. In the book *The Hidden Lamp*, Joan Sutherland commented that Lingzhao's action

obliterates the idea that there is a helper and a helped. Compassion isn't a commodity we deliver but a commitment to help liberate the intimacy already inherent in any situation. . . . Usually the most intimate response to another's difficulty begins with the willingness not to flee. Fleeing can take the form of abandoning the situation, and it can also mean escaping into 'helping,' into a whole constellation of ideas about what ought to happen. Intimacy is being willing to stay and accompany and listen, to be vulnerable and surprised and flexible. It's a willingness to fall with someone else, and see what becomes possible when we do.[11]

And why did Layman Pang respond by saying "luckily no one was looking"? Although on first glance, it seems to suggest that he was worried about someone else frowning upon them, I think his remark is to alert us to the internalized "someone else"—that is, our inner critic—our tendency to question whether we have done a good job, to judge whether we have done enough, and to chastise ourselves when we think we have done something wrong. It reminds me that before we can truly serve others, we need to be compassionate towards ourselves. It reminds me that even with my imperfections, failures, and disappointments, I can still incline my body, heart, and mind toward loving-kindness and compassion for all beings, including myself. Compassion is the expression of our innermost nature. We make a commitment, and we inevitably fall off the track, but, with determination, we renew our commitment. The coming back again and again is the practice. The act of returning is the practice of compassion.

In closing, I would like to share with you a *mettā* practice written by the Buddhist teacher Larry Yang that I found to be particularly inspiring.[12] I hope it will inspire you, too.

> May I be loving, open, and aware in this moment;
> If I cannot be loving, open, and aware in this moment, may
>   I be kind;
> If I cannot be kind, may I be non-judgmental;
> If I cannot be non-judgmental, may I not cause harm;
> If I cannot not cause harm, may I cause the least harm possible.

References

1. Williams M, Penman D. *Mindfulness: An Eight-Week Plan for Finding Peace in a Frantic World.* Emmaus, PA: Rodale Books; 2012.
2. Thich Nhat Hahn. *Reconciliation: Healing The Inner Child.* Berkeley, CA: Parallax Press; 2010.
3. Van Gennep A. *The Rites of Passage.* Chicago: University of Chicago Press; 1960.
4. Douglas M. *Purity and Danger: An Analysis of Concepts of Pollution and Taboo.* New York: Routledge; 1966.
5. Glassman B, Fields R. *Instructions to the Cook: A Zen Master's Lessons in Living a Life That Matters.* New York: Bell Tower; 2013.
6. Halifax J. *Being with Dying: Cultivating Compassion and Fearlessness in the Presence of Death.* Boston, MA: Shambhala; 2009.

7. Monnett M. Developing a Buddhist approach to pastoral care: A peacemaker's view. *J Pastoral Care Counsel.* 2005;59:57–61.

8. Kleinman A, Eisenberg L, Good B. Culture, illness, and care. *Ann Intern Med.* 1978;88:252–258.

9. West CP, Dyrbye LN, Erwin PJ, Shanafelt TD. Interventions to prevent and reduce physician burnout: A systematic review and meta-analysis. *Lancet.* 2016;388(10057):2272–2281.

10. Panagioti M, Panagopoulou E, Bower P, et al. Controlled interventions to reduce burnout in physicians: A systematic review and meta-analysis. *JAMA Intern Med.* 2017;177(2):195–205.

11. Sutherland J. Lingzhao's helping. In: Caplow ZF, Moon RS, eds. *The Hidden Lamp: Stories from Twenty-Five Centuries of Awakened Women.* Boston, MA: Wisdom Publications; 2013:293–295.

12. Yang L. In the moments of non-awakening. In: Melvin McLeod, Tynette Deveaux, ed. *Buddhadharma: The Practitioner's Quarterly.* Boulder, CO: Shambhala Publications; 2019:87–95.

Acknowledgements

Writing this book has been a labour of love, and it would not have been possible without the guidance and support of many teachers, friends, and family. While it is impossible to list them all here, I especially want to offer my deepest gratitude to a number of people.

I am deeply indebted to my teacher, Roshi Joan Halifax. Thank you for finding me when I was about to withdraw from medicine. Your wise, intimate, and caring counsel has accompanied me through the challenging yet transformative "margin" stage of my journey. I can still hear your words, always encouraging me to draw on my experience to serve clinicians, as there is so much struggle, distress, and burnout in healthcare. I hope I have understood, carried, and disseminated your teachings authentically in these pages to benefit many more beings.

My great thanks to the Upaya chaplaincy program and the many teachers involved—Sensei Hozan Alan Senauke, Sensei Joshin Byrnes, Sensei Petra Zenryū Hubbeling, and Rev. Michelle Nicole. I have learned so much from the training, which I hope you can see permeating the pages in this book. You have trained many modern-day bodhisattvas to carry out the much needed work in this world.

I am deeply grateful to my chaplaincy mentor, Rev. Marilyn Whitney. You have patiently, diligently, and thoughtfully read and commented on every one of the papers and the thesis that I wrote, which combined to total more than 350 pages! I thank you for sharing your wealth of experience, steadfast support, and spiritual friendship so that I can become a better chaplain and a more spiritually matured being.

I am forever indebted to my counsellor, Len Choptiany. You have been a staunch supporter, sounding board, and trusted confidant throughout the whole writing process and beyond. I thank you for your deep insight, humour, and the many thought-provoking conversations that we shared. I cherish the many dialogs we had—from philosophy, psychology, spirituality, to my inner conflicts, trials, and tribulations, and to the joy, peace, and transformation that I have experienced.

I look forward to many more stimulating discussions with you. Most of all, thank you for teaching me to be genuine and authentic despite the "noise" in this world.

I also want to express my deepest gratitude to my local mentor and friend, Rev. Andrew Blake. Thank you for being you and for allowing me to work alongside you in the Mindfulness and Compassion Training for Health and End-of-Life Care Professionals program. I would not have appreciated, at the deepest level, the personal struggles and system challenges that healthcare workers face without working with you in this program. You have helped me to assimilate what I have learned and apply it in the real world. You and your wife, Rev. Angie Blake, have shown me what deep healing looks like, especially in difficult times. I am indebted to both you and Angie for helping me to deepen my practice through your tireless effort to build a nurturing and supportive local *sangha*. I look forward to spending more time with you and the *sangha* in the beautiful, serene, and sacred Sarana Springs!

My great thanks to Dr. Nicholas Wang, Dr. Michael Roberts, and Michael Apollo for reading previous drafts of the book. Your enthusiastic, candid, and critical comments have propelled me to the finishing line. I treasure our dharma friendships as a fellow sojourner on this path. I also want to thank Professor Terri Lewis, Rosanne Steinbach, and Dr. Peter Karagiannis for your constructive feedback on the book. Thanks also goes to Mano Chandrakumar for your technical support and, more importantly, your patience, friendship, and encouragement over the past many years.

My deep gratitude to my editor, Marta Moldvai, for believing in this project right from the start. You, and the anonymous reviewers, have helped push my envelope to not be afraid to share my personal observations and experiences and to share my heart with the readers. The book would not have come across in the same way without your astute input, nor would it be as fulfilling to write without being able to express fully what I really want to convey. I also thank Dr. Stephen Post for your encouragement, guidance, and enthusiasm on this book.

Thanks to my sons, James and Stephen, for keeping your noise level down while I worked on a major portion of this book at home during the social distancing period of the covid-19 pandemic. Both of you have given me so much fun, joy, and love in my life. I'd love to hear what you think of the messages of the book when you grow up! I hope that we, and especially your generation and those after you, will come out of the pandemic and work toward a more compassionate, just, and inclusive world.

Finally, to my beloved husband, friend, and confidant, Bill. I would not be who I am today without your patience, trust, and love. Thanks for being there for me in good times and bad, for never doubting my ability, and for bringing out the best in me.

Resources

Currently Available Compassion-Based Trainings/ Interventions

Here is a list of programs with information on their targeted populations, original formats, and developers. Many programs are now offered in a variety of formats and at multiple locations. Please check the corresponding website for latest information.

Being with Dying: Professional Training Program for Clinicians in Compassionate Care of the Seriously Ill and Dying

- Website: https://www.upaya.org/being-with-dying/
- Targeted population: Healthcare professionals
- Format: 7 all-day in-person group sessions
- Developer: Joan Halifax, PhD, at Upaya Institute and Zen Center

Cognitively Based Compassion Training (CBCT)

- Website: https://www.compassion.emory.edu/cbct-compassion-training/index.html
- Targeted population: General public, healthcare professionals, educators
- Format: 8 weekly (2-hour) in-person group sessions (intensive trainings now available)
- Developer: Lobsang Tenzin Negi, PhD, at Emory University

Compassion Cultivation Training

- Website: https://www.compassioninstitute.com/the-program/ compassion-cultivation-training/ and http://ccare.stanford.edu/ education/about-compassion-training/
- Targeted population: General public, healthcare professionals, and some clinical populations
- Format: 8 weekly (2-hour) in-person group sessions and daily meditation practices
- Developer: Thupten Jinpa, PhD, at Stanford University

Compassion-Focused Therapy

- Website: https://www.compassionatemind.co.uk/
- Targeted population: Clinical populations (chronic and complex mental health problems with high levels of shame and self-criticism, often from abusive backgrounds)
- Format:
  - Individual therapy
  - In-person group (Compassionate Mind Training): 8 to 12 weekly (2-hour) sessions
- Developer: Paul Gilbert, PhD

Cultivating Emotional Balance (CEB)

- Website: https://cultivating-emotional-balance.org/about/
- Targeted population: General public
- Format: 8 weeks (4 all-day and 4 evening) in-person group sessions (online format now available)
- Developers: Paul Ekman, PhD, Alan Wallace, PhD, and Mind and Life Institute

G.R.A.C.E.: Training in Cultivating
Compassion-Based Interactions

- Website: https://www.upaya.org/program/g-r-a-c-e-training-in-cultivating-compassion-based-interactions-2021/?id=2318
- Targeted population: Healthcare professionals and general public
- Format: 2 all-day in-person group sessions
- Developers: Joan Halifax, PhD, Tony Back, MD, and Cynda Hylton Rushton, PhD, RN

Mindfulness and Compassion Certificate Training
Program for Health and End-of-Life Care Professionals

- Website: http://www.saranainstitute.org/mc-training/
- Targeted population: Healthcare professionals
- Format: 10 all-day in-person group sessions over 9 months
- Developer: Rev. Andrew Blake

Mindful Self-Compassion

- Website: https://centerformsc.org/all-cmsc-offerings/
- Targeted population: General public and some clinical populations
- Format: 8 weekly (2.75-hour) in-person group sessions plus a half-day retreat (intensive trainings and online format now available)
- Developers: Kristen Neff, PhD, and Christopher Germer, PhD

Further Reading

- Armstrong K. *Twelve Steps to a Compassionate Life*. New York: Alfred A. Knopf; 2010.
- Beltzner E. *How to Tame the Tumbles: The Mindful Self-Compassionate Way*. Ontario: Mosaic Press; 2019.

- Brach T. *Radical Acceptance: Embracing Your Life with the Heart of a Buddha*. New York: Bantam Dell; 2003.
- Brach T. *Radical Compassion: Learning to Love Yourself and Your World with the Practice of RAIN*. New York: Viking; 2019.
- Brown B. *Soul Without Shame: A Guide to Liberating Yourself from the Judge Within*. Boston, MA: Shambhala Publications; 1998.
- Brown B. *The Gifts of Imperfection: Let Go of Who You Think You're Supposed to Be and Embrace Who You Are*. Center City, MN: Hazelden; 2010.
- Campbell J. *The Hero with a Thousand Faces*. Novato, CA: New World Library; 2008.
- Chokyi Nyima Rinpoche, Shlim DR. *Medicine and Compassion: A Tibetan Lama's Guidance for Caregivers*. Boston, MA: Wisdom Publications; 2004.
- Dalai Lama HH, Cutler HC. *The Art of Happiness: A Handbook for Living*. New York: Penguin Group; 1998.
- Dalai Lama HH. *Ethics for the New Millennium*. New York: Riverhead Books; 1999.
- Dalai Lama HH. *Transforming the Mind: Teachings on Generating Compassion*. London: Thorsons; 2000.
- Dalai Lama HH, Tutu D, Abrams D. *The Book of Joy: Lasting Happiness in a Changing World*. New York: Avery; 2016.
- Epstein R. *Attending: Medicine, Mindfulness, and Humanity*. New York: Scribner; 2017.
- Germer C. *The Mindful Path to Self-Compassion: Freeing Yourself from Destructive Thoughts and Emotions*. New York: Guilford Press; 2009.
- Germer CK, Siegel RD. *Wisdom and Compassion in Psychotherapy: Deepening Mindfulness in Clinical Practice*. New York: Guilford Press; 2012.
- Gilbert P. *The Compassionate Mind*. London: Constable & Robinson; 2009.
- Giles CA, Miller WB, eds. *The Arts of Contemplative Care: Pioneering Voices in Buddhist Chaplaincy and Pastoral Work*. Boston, MA: Wisdom Publications; 2012.
- Goldstein J, Kornfield J. *Seeking the Heart of Wisdom: The Path of Insight Meditation*. Boston, MA: Shambhala Publications; 1987.
- Goleman D, Davidson RJ. *Altered Traits: Science Reveals How Meditation Changes Your Mind, Brain, and Body*. New York: Penguin Random House; 2017.
- Halifax J. *Being with Dying: Cultivating Compassion and Fearlessness in the Presence of Death*. Boston, MA: Shambhala; 2009.
- Halifax J. *Standing at the Edge*. New York: Martin's Press; 2018.
- Jinpa T. *A Fearless Heart: How the Courage to Be Compassionate Can Transform Our Lives*. New York: Hudson Street Press; 2015.
- King MLJ. *Strength to Love*. Boston, MA: Beacon Press; 2019.
- Kabat-Zinn J. *Wherever You Go, There You Are: Mindfulness Meditation in Everyday Life*. New York: Hyperion; 1994.
- Kornfield J. *A Path with Heart*. New York: Bantam Books; 1993.

- Lown B. *The Lost Art of Healing: Practicing Compassion in Medicine.* New York: Ballantine Books; 1999.
- Macy J. *World as Lover, World as Self: A Guide to Living Fully in Turbulent Times.* Berkeley, CA: Parallax Press; 2003.
- Maull F. *Radical Responsibility: How to Move Beyond Blame, Fearlessly Live Your Highest Purpose, and Become an Unstoppable Force for Good.* Boulder, CO: Sounds True; 2019.
- Neff K. *Self-Compassion: The Proven Power of Being Kind to Yourself.* New York: William Morrow; 2015.
- Rosenberg MB. *Nonviolent Communication: A Language of Life.* Encinitas, CA: PuddleDancer Press; 2003.
- Salzberg S. *Lovingkindness: The Revolutionary Art of Happiness.* Boston, MA: Shambhala Publications, Inc; 1995.
- Salzberg S. *The Force of Kindness: Change Your Life with Love and Compassion.* Boulder, CO: Sounds True; 2005.
- Siegel DJ. *Mind: A Journey to the Heart of Being Human.* New York: W. W. Norton & Company; 2016.
- Sofer OJ. *Say What You Mean: A Mindful Approach to Nonviolent Communication.* Boulder, CO: Shambhala Publications; 2018.
- Sogyal Rinpoche. *The Tibetan Book of Living and Dying: New Spiritual Classic from One of the Foremost Interpreters of Tibetan Buddhism.* San Francisco, CA: HarperOne; 1992.
- Tsabary S. *The Conscious Parent: Transforming Ourselves, Empowering Our Children.* Vancouver: Namaste Publishing; 2010.
- Thich Nhat Hahn. *Peace Is Every Step: The Path of Mindfulness in Everyday Life.* New York: Bantam Books; 1991.
- Thich Nhat Hanh. *Teachings on Love.* Berkeley, CA: Parallax Press; 1997.
- Thich Nhat Hahn. *Reconciliation: Healing the Inner Child.* Berkeley, CA: Parallax Press; 2010.
- Thich Nhat Hahn. *No Mud, No Lotus: The Art of Transforming Suffering.* Berkeley, CA: Parallax Press; 2014.
- Tolle E. *The Power of Now: A Guide to Spiritual Enlightenment.* Novato, CA: New World Library; 1999.
- Tolle E. *A New Earth: Awakening to Your Life's Purpose.* New York: Dutton; 2005.
- Trzeciak S, Mazzarelli A. *Compassionomics: The Revolutionary Scientific Evidence That Caring Makes a Difference.* Pensacola, FL: Studer Group, LLC; 2019.
- Treleaven DA. *Trauma-Sensitive Mindfulness: Practices for Safe and Transformative Healing.* New York: W.W. Norton & Company; 2018.
- Tutu D. *No Future Without Forgiveness.* New York: Doubleday; 1999.
- Weller F. *The Wild Edge of Sorrow: Rituals of Renewal and the Sacred Work of Grief.* Berkeley, CA: North Atlantic Books; 2015.
- Williams M, Penman D. *Mindfulness: An Eight-Week Plan for Finding Peace in a Frantic World.* Emmaus, PA: Rodale Books; 2012.

General Websites on Mindfulness and Compassion

- A Mindful Society: https://amindfulsociety.org/
- Awareness in Action: www.awarenessinaction.org
- The Center for Compassion and Altruism Research and Education: http://ccare.stanford.edu/
- The Center for Contemplative Mind in Society: www.contemplativemind.org
- The Center for Healthy Minds: www.centerhealthyminds.org
- The Center for Nonviolent Communication: www.cnvc.org
- Centre for Mindfulness Research and Practice: www.bangor.ac.uk/mindfulness
- The Centre for Mindfulness Studies: https://www.mindfulnessstudies.com/
- The Charter for Compassion: www.charterforcompassion.org
- Compassionate Living: www.compassionateliving.info
- Christopher Germer: www.mindfulselfcompassion.org
- The Compassion Institute: www.compassioninstitute.com
- The Compassionate Mind Foundation: www.compassionatemind.co.uk
- Foundation for Active Compassion: www.foundationforactivecompassion.org/
- Greater Good: The Science of a Meaningful Life: www.greatergood.berkeley.edu
- Institute for Meditation and Psychotherapy: www.meditationandpsychotherapy.org
- Mindful website: www.mindful.org
- Mindful Awareness Research Center at University of California Los Angeles: www.marc.ucla.edu
- Mindfulness Exercises: www.mindfulnessexercises.com
- The Mindfulness Institute: www.mindfulnessinstitute.ca
- Mindfulness page maintained by David Fresco: www.personal.kent.edu/%7Edfresco/mindfulness.htm
- Mindfulness page maintained by Christopher Walsh: www.mindfulness.org.au
- Mindfulness Research Guide: www.goamra.org
- Mind and Life Institute: www.mindandlife.org
- Mindsight Institute: www.mindsightinstitute.com
- Plum Village: https://plumvillage.org/
- Sarana Institute: http://www.saranainstitute.org/
- University of California at San Diego Center for Mindfulness: mindfulness.ucsd.edu/
- University of Massachusetts Center for Mindfulness: www.umassmed.edu/cfm/index.aspx
- Upaya Institute and Zen Center: https://www.upaya.org/
- The Wellspring Institute for Neuroscience and Contemplative Wisdom: www.wisebrain.org

About the Author

Agnes M.F. Wong, MD, PhD, FRCSC, is Professor of Ophthalmology, Neurology, and Psychology at the University of Toronto and an active staff ophthalmologist at The Hospital for Sick Children in Toronto. Born and raised in Hong Kong, Dr. Wong received her Bachelor of Arts degree in Psychology and Biology from Boston University, Doctor of Medicine degree from McGill University, and Doctor of Philosophy degree in Neuroscience from the University of Toronto. Her clinical training included an Ophthalmology residency and a Neuro-Ophthalmology fellowship at the University of Toronto, and a Pediatric Ophthalmology and Strabismus fellowship at Washington University in St. Louis.

Dr. Wong is the former Ophthalmologist-in-Chief at The Hospital for Sick Children. She is also the former Vice Chair of Research in the Department of Ophthalmology at the University of Toronto, where she held the inaugural John and Melinda Thompson Chair in Vision Neuroscience for 10 years. In her career as a physician-scientist, Dr. Wong has published extensively in the field of ophthalmology and vision sciences, including the textbook *Eye Movement Disorders*, also published by Oxford University Press. Dr. Wong has travelled widely as a visiting professor, is a much sought-after invited speaker, and has won many research and teaching awards nationally and internationally.

Dr. Wong completed chaplaincy training with Roshi Joan Halifax at the Upaya Zen Center in Santa Fe, New Mexico, USA. She also completed the Mindfulness-Based Cognitive Therapy Teacher Training Intensive. She is a facilitator in the Mindfulness and Compassion Training for Health and End-of-Life Care Professionals program at the Sarana Institute in Toronto. Her current ministry includes prison and end-of-life care. She also focuses on physician wellness by integrating mindfulness, compassion, reflective practice, and system thinking as tools for physicians to enhance their own well-being and to improve the healthcare system.

Dr. Wong lives in Toronto with her husband, Bill Webb, and two sons, James and Stephen.

Index